Stolen Memories

Stolen Memories

One Family's Experience With Alzheimer's Disease

Marie Cloud

Writers Club Press
San Jose New York Lincoln Shanghai

Stolen Memories
One Family's Experience With Alzheimer's Disease

Writers Club Press
an imprint of iUniverse.com, Inc.

For information address:
iUniverse.com, Inc.
5220 S 16th, Ste. 200
Lincoln, NE 68512
www.iuniverse.com

ISBN: 0-595-15849-8

Printed in the United States of America

DEDICATION

This book is dedicated to my loving mother and father. I thank my wonderful husband, children, grandchild who gave me support and strength to write this book. Also I would like to thank my brother, his wife and family for all they did for my mother. If not for the continued encouragement and support from my mother-in-law I am not sure this book would have ever been completed.

ACKNOWLEDGMENTS

John Mudge
Peggy Lambert
All of the women from the WWW, writers group

INTRODUCTION

This is a story about how Alzheimer disease (AD) affected our family. It touches upon the guilt and confusion that can result from being a caregiver to a parent with Alzheimer's disease. It describes how trying to separate the words of an AD patient from those of a parent, can create many problems for the caregiver. My husband and I spent far too long denying that my mother had this disease. This book explains the difficulties we faced in coping with my mother's illness. It is **not** a story of what we did right, it is a story of what we could have done better.

My mother lived with us for more than fifteen years and helped raise our children. This story shows the contrast between my mother's life before the disease, and what happened to all of us as a result of her developing Alzheimer's disease. As many Baby-Boomers reach the age of fifty, more research is vital. As this quotation from the Alzheimer Association Web Page states: "At some point, persons with AD will require 24-hour care, including assistance with daily activities such as eating, grooming and toileting. The financing of care for AD including costs of diagnosis, treatment, nursing home care and formal or paid care—is estimated to be more than $100 billion each year. The federal government covers $4.0 billion and the states another $4.1 billion. Much of the remaining costs are borne by the patients and their families."

During my mother's life, she often told me that she worked and saved so she could leave money to her family when she died. This did not happen. Of course she left something much more precious than money. She left her love and wonderful memories. Before she died, the Alzheimer care facilities absorbed nearly everything she saved. This is not unusual at all. It happens every day. I often wonder what happens to those who are too poor to contribute their retirement and do not have savings to pay these fees.

STOLEN MEMORIES is a tool to help others recognize and come to grips with the disease sooner than we did. This book addresses several important issues, such as what this disease can do to a family, how relationships can affect being a caregiver for an AD patient, and the difficulties of an untrained caregiver attempting to manage an AD family member.

A caregiver needs to understand the different aspects of any disease. Without specific knowledge about their loved one's disease, a family member acting as a caregiver can easily be overwhelmed with guilt and depression.

To any family members who are caregiving an Alzheimer patient, please get help. Do not try to do it alone. Attend support groups. Read as much as possible about the disease. Take breaks from the patient now and then. My husband and I did not do enough of these things and it nearly destroyed us and did not help my mother.

PART I

CHANGING TIMES

CHAPTER 1

"It can't be true." I held the letter from the psychiatrist in my shaking hand.

"Well, we had to find out. Now that we know, we can deal with it," Joe said.

"You're right. We've been fighting something unknown for too long. It's just been too hard for me to admit the truth." I looked into his sad eyes. "My God, you've read the books about Alzheimer's disease. I don't know if I can watch this happen to her? It's just not fair." My muffled words filled Joe's shoulder. For the last year our means of communication about my mother was behind the closed door of our bedroom while she slept.

"We'll get through it together." Joe rubbed my back trying to calm me down.

"She never did anything to deserve this horrible disease." I tried to keep my voice low.

This had been just another tumultuous day, one of many over the past year and a half. It made me sick to see Alzheimer's disease steal away my mother's mind and her once so vital life. This intelligent woman once filled with energy now did not know when to shower. I resented the toll that this terrible disease had taken on all of us. After seeing the devastating effects on Mom's mind thus far, I could not imagine what the future held.

As usual my husband Joe comforted me. He told me that I was not alone, but I felt alone. She was my mother, I was losing her day by day, and I could do nothing to stop this thing.

Since no single clinical test exists to identify Alzheimer's disease, we followed the procedures suggested by her general practitioner. Prior to her visit to the psychiatrist, Mom's doctor ran a battery of tests and gave her a complete physical exam. He requested an analysis of her blood and urine, chest x-rays, and an electrocardiogram. From the beginning of her memory problems, her doctor referred to her disease as some type of dementia. I knew about dementia but I did not know much about Alzheimer's disease at that point. The little I did know scared me so much that I could not admit this might be what she had.

After her physical, her doctor asked me to document her behavior during the following week. I did not have time to write a journal, but I took a few notes every day for a week on her unusual behavior. I had no problem preparing a list.

- She was unable to form words.
- We had to monitor her eating habits because she put strange combinations of food such as cottage cheese with ground beef and sauerkraut together.
- She could no longer maintain a checkbook or pay her bills.
- We had to take her car keys away from her because she had become a danger to herself and others.
- She repeatedly asked the same question.

Every week Mom wanted me to take her to the dentist because she said that she had too much saliva in her mouth. Her dentist, bless his heart, was so patient with her. He ran a suction device around inside her mouth and rubbed a cleaning tool over her teeth. It only took a few minutes but he was extremely kind to her. Her general practitioner had never seen this symptom, but I have a strong feeling it was somehow related to the disease. She continued having this complaint until she went to the next, even worse level.

Mom also constantly lost her belongings. Every day we searched for her purse, shoes, clothing, and even her teeth. We found her teeth in her purse and her purse behind the bathroom door or under her clothes.

One day while she was still asleep, I got up early to shovel snow off the driveway. When Mom awoke, she came outside in 30-degree temperature, wearing only a light, housedress and sandals with no socks. Since my back was turned to her, I had no idea how long she had been outside before I saw her. As soon as I did, I took her inside and dressed her appropriately.

I called Mom's doctor to give him the list. He asked me to set up an appointment with a psychiatrist who specialized in memory problems and dementia. My mother fought us all the way. Mom wanting no part of this exam. She still had moments of lucidity when she knew something was going very wrong with her and became fearful even with her familiar family doctor. Now we were taking her to this strange doctor, and she wanted to know why.

As I opened the car door at the doctor's office, she looked at me with an angry look in her eyes and said, "You want to put me away, don't you?" My head began to spin from guilt. She had a way of doing that to me.

I held her hand, looked into her eyes and said, "We just want to see if the doctor can help you feel better and maybe find a way to help you do the things you used to enjoy." I could tell she did not believe a word of it or perhaps did not understand.

Luckily the doctor was pleasant and knew how to put her at ease. Mom began to relax as he asked her questions. I could not believe how much she remembered about math and numbers. Nevertheless, when he asked simple questions like her middle name and if she had children or grandchildren, she did not know. She agreed to the doctor's suggestion that I wait in the other room for her. He then conducted neurological and mental status assessments. He also conducted neuropsychological testing that measures psychological observations on behavior and the mind as well as neurological observations on the brain and nervous system.

In the waiting room, I began reading a pamphlet about different types of dementia. When I glanced at the one on Alzheimer's disease, I gasped in fear. I knew after reading the symptoms this must be what she had. Everything in the book put out by the Alzheimer's Association fit her behavior perfectly. It said, "The symptoms included gradual memory loss, decline in the ability to perform routine tasks, disorientation, difficulty in learning, loss of language skills, impairment of judgment and planning, and personality changes." I learned that while the rate of progression is different with each individual, and can take from three to twenty years, the average length of time between the start of the disease's symptoms until death is eight years. It also said that Alzheimer's patients eventually are unable to care for themselves.

I became more horrified with each page I read. I handed the pamphlet to Joe and we both cringed at the turn our future had just taken. The remainder of our time in the waiting room was spent in shock. Neither of us wanted to believe how closely the symptoms in the book matched Mom's. When we returned home that day, I called the Alzheimer's Association and requested that they send the literature to me at work. I did not want Mom to find them and in a lucid moment think the worst.

Unfortunately, there was not a way for the doctors to really confirm a diagnosis of Alzheimer's disease. This frustrated me even more. At least we had done everything we could to rule out other, curable diseases. That knowledge helped a little.

During the ten days between her test and the diagnosis, I felt like I was hanging from a skyscraper by a rubber band. I knew but did not want to believe the truth. I hoped to be told she had a curable disease, anything other than Alzheimer's disease.

Then the results came in the mail. Since I was the first one home, I held my breath as opened the letter from the Psychiatrist. As I read the results, I felt that rubber band break and I plunged into a despair that I did not come out of it for several years. I knew I would be sitting idly by watching my mother lose all that was so important to her. The mother I once knew would become a shell of the woman who raised me. I did not know if I had the strength to watch her go through this.

Joe and I climbed into bed. He tried to comfort me but I moved to the other side of the bed. He wanted to help me but I also knew it was up to me. I was responsible. How would I deal with this? I drifted into the past, to the days when Mom was a woman ahead of her time. I tried to remember how things were long ago. I needed to remember the strength she had during those times to get through this.

*   *   *

My father had been in the Air Force for twenty-one years. I came into the world in Pennsylvania and my brother Robert was born in Texas. In 1955 we moved to Germany for three and a half years. When I started high school in 1960 in Washington, D.C., they transferred my father to a remote Italian air force base. This left my mother behind for a year and a half to take care of me and my brother, the house, the finances, and her full-time job. He hated to leave but together they decided that doing that was best for the family. They did not want to uproot us to take another assignment during my high school years. I did not realize until later just what a sacrifice they made for me.

I remember one summer when my mother's boss hired me to clean the three offices where she worked. Her boss enjoyed helping young people and the job gave me the chance to be productive. While I cleaned, I watched my mother. She was so organized and intelligent. I waited for her fingers to catch fire as she typed and asked her how many words she typed a minute. In a meek voice she said, "Oh, about a hundred and twenty." My mouth dropped open. I could barely type thirty-five words a minute without errors.

Mom did not like to show it, but she was a very independent woman. She had always excelled in school. I was only an average student. This and many other things in my life had given me low self-esteem, which is why I related more to my father. He had never been a good student either, and later I could see that he often felt he was not good enough for Mom. My mother and I saw things about him that he did not. He could speak fluently in several languages and could charm anyone within a few minutes. I knew Mom saw those things long before I did, and that is why she fell in love with him all those years ago.

*   *   *

When I woke up that January day in 1993, after receiving the results from the psychiatrist, I began to prepare for the unknown road that lay ahead. We could no longer leave Mom alone for fear she might take off and not find her way home or leave the stove burners turned on. I was glad I worked a twelve-hour shift. I worked six hours on Wednesdays then twelve hours from Thursdays through Saturdays, which meant I had more time to spend at home with my mother. It helped that Joe worked a regular nine-to-five shift Monday through Friday so he could watch over Mom on the weekends.

I was not sure where to start looking for a day-care place for Mom but I needed a safe place for her to stay while Joe and I worked. Finding Neighborhood House took me about eight phone calls. I started by calling the Alzheimer's Association. They transferred me here and there until I finally talked to someone who referred me to the Catholic Archdiocese. After being connected to several different areas, I received the name and phone number for Neighborhood House. Lynn, the manager of the Neighborhood House nearest to us was very helpful. She told me how I should handle Mom's acclimation, what and how they charge, and the times to drop her off and pick her up. They even had a bus with limited service, but it did not go as far as our home.

After talking to Lynn, I realized I needed to take a week's vacation to obtain and prepare the necessary paperwork to enroll my mother. I hated to take a week off in January, I was afraid that I would need more time off later to care for Mom, but I had no choice. Her general practitioner and psychiatrist had to fill out forms regarding her condition. I had to provide information so that the caregivers would be aware of Mom's food likes and dislikes, any fears she had, and which medicines she took.

Neighborhood House charged by the amount the person could afford to pay. This meant I needed to obtain all the information about her Social Security and Retirement benefits. Her once perfectly organized records had become a large garbage bag with everything thrown in together. It broke my heart as I searched through the bag. She hated for anyone to touch her papers. When I had to look for anything, she said, "Don't do that. Those are mine. You can't have them." She looked at me with pure hatred in her eyes. I made it a point never to go into her room or her through her things unless I had no choice.

Once I had enrolled her at Neighborhood House, I worried about Mom's reaction. With Lynn's help, my mother felt right at home. Lynn asked her to "help" the older patients. Mom did not totally understand and at times became leery, but overall she seemed to enjoy being there. I stayed with her for the entire first day to help adjust her into her new environment. For the next two days, I returned or called several times during the day to make sure she was doing okay. They kept her so busy that after only three days I could leave her alone. After a week, she actually looked forward to going, but I always felt guilty leaving her there. I do not know why because they took great care of her. It seemed our roles were reversed now; I was her mother and she was my child.

At the end of the week, Lynn told me that my mother already knew her favorite activities. Mom loved their walks, but Lynn said they had to watch her because she wandered. She seemed to enjoy it when they brought in baby animals and she liked doing simple crafts, but she had to have a day-care worker help her put them together. I knew she required help with crafts. For Christmas I bought her some simple coloring and pasting crafts for ages three to eight. I hoped that she could stay busy doing crafts while I did my housework and laundry. But it did not work out because I had to sit with her and show her how to do even those simple tasks. Mom just could not remember what to do minutes after I explained the instructions to her. Lynn said to have one of their workers constantly going around the table helping each person, made it easier to keep her interest. She explained that Alzheimer's patients needed constant prodding to do tasks.

Day-care had been good for my mother and for me. I was finally able to think at work again, knowing that she was in good hands. I still had stress but Joe and I had a few other moments to live our life. We knew we had done a good thing by finding Neighborhood House.

When she returned home after her time at day-care, our evening rituals remained the same as before. Mom was more comfortable knowing what would happen. She did not like a lot of changes. So after dinner and her shower, I helped Mom put the videotape into the VCR in her room. For years she loved to work in her garden during the day and taped the soap operas to watch in her room at night. I think observing her trying to use her VCR showed the clearest deterioration of her memory. Because she did this every day, it was a means of monitoring how her mind was working. I remember that before the onset of Alzheimer's disease, she could follow the directions to record her programs. In a two-year period, she could do less and less. Since the beginning of the summer, I began doing more of the processes for her. Now I had to do everything from putting the tape into the VCR to hitting "Play" and "Stop." I had to go in and see whether the programs were over or not. Occasionally I went in to find her staring at a blank screen. I was not even sure if she knew what she was watching.

CHAPTER 2

It was only a weeks into January 1993. Each day seemed to run together. Everything stayed the same. On my days off, Mom expected me to cater to her every whim. Whenever she wanted to go to the foot doctor or the dentist, I had to drop what I was doing and go. She insisted I take her for walks or sit and do crafts with her. Her demands were like those of a spoiled child. I guess since the day-care place kept her so busy, she came to expect the same things at home.

Nights had become very difficult because she did not sleep well. There were nights she woke up screaming. Other nights she wandered throughout the house. Joe and I never had enough sleep. We worried about her leaving the house and taking off or falling down the stairs and hurting herself.

One day I became sick with stomach flu that was going around at work. Being in bed for the day was a rarity for me. I fought illness and hated being laid up. It also did not sit well with my mother. She did not understand why I was not with her.

Joe came home from work when he realized how sick I was. He knew I could not watch out for my mother properly. Before he arrived home, Mom kept coming into my room and asking me to do things for her. She did not understand why I was not paying more attention to her. I told her repeatedly that I was sick. Finally Joe came home. He could see things were not going well. Mom started asking him why I was staying in the bedroom. He decided to let her help in some way and asked Mom to bring me some crackers on a tray.

I will never forget that day as long as I live. Standing at the foot of my bed and holding a tray, she said, "You know I like you today, not like the other days. I usually don't like you." When she walked out of the room, I felt like I was falling into a deep well. My head was spinning, my mind careening out of control. My pillow, already wet from perspiration, now was saturated with tears. I knew in my head that this was the disease talking, but I wondered if deep down my mother really felt that way. Was I truly a disappointment to her?

I fell back to sleep feeling even more sick than before and deeply saddened by my mother's comments. The flu and stress had taken their toll on me, but the worst part of that day was to last a long time—reliving my mother's words over and over in my head. It almost killed me to find out how she felt. I loved and respected her so much my whole life. Now I felt she did not love me, and that I was indeed a disappointment to her.

The most difficult part of the disease for me was that I could never separate the disease from my mother. When she spoke angry words, I felt like a child being punished. Her words hit me like knives in the chest. I tried so hard to please her, to make up for any ill feelings I ever had toward her, but I knew this disease would not give me the time I needed. It was too late. As I remembered our past, my head began to throb.

* * *

I had two failed marriages. It seemed for many years I could not succeed at anything I did. I often felt like a failure.

Mom, on the other hand, was always there. She had two children, kept a full-time job, and took care of all the finances and books for the household. It seemed to me that she could do anything. My mother,

Rose, was a very special woman. She had been through very difficult times as a child. She was the oldest of five children. Just after her youngest sister was born, her father had died, leaving her mother to raise all five children alone. Times were tough for everyone then. The depression left many without money or work. Mary, her mother, my grandmother, had a job with the federal government as a secretary. Mary counted on Mom to help and placed many responsibilities upon her shoulders. Mary's mother eventually came to live with them and helped watch the children while she went out to work to try to survive. Now Mom would do the same thing for me. Her life seemed to have come full circle. After my father died and my divorce was finalized, my mother came to help me with my children.

My first marriage had been a mistake. I had married too young and we divorced in a year. Mom and Dad stood by me after that marriage and helped me get on my feet again. I went home to live and began trying to rebuild my life. Unfortunately, I seemed destined to repeat the same mistakes. I remarried in a year. Mom and Dad tried to lend me support but I always felt I needed to get out on my own. It just was not right for me to be living at home with them. Perhaps that was why I remarried so soon after my divorce.

My second husband, Fred, and I lived in Maryland in a large, white brick house with our perfect little daughter Tonya. I should have been happy. Financially we were in good shape but problems existed in our marriage. Looking back on it, I realize that my way of finding happiness was to have children. Since Tonya gave me purpose, I thought having more children might make me happier. Once she started going to school full-time, I began feeling sad. Even going out to work everyday did not help. I had been unable to conceive a second child for five years and that did not help. I knew Fred did not care and do not think he ever wanted any more children. I did but felt I was a failure because I could not get pregnant.

After seven years, I found out I was pregnant. I put aside my fears about Fred and his drinking for the joy of being a mother again. After all, most of the time things were okay. He adored our daughter and never physically hurt me. He had a way of making me feel worthless, but I thought I could handle that. After all in the early 70's women were less likely to complain.

During the fifth month of pregnancy, I started spotting and nearly lost the baby. No one will ever know how much carrying my baby meant to me. This baby defined me as a person. I know now that it should not have been that way. I know that was no reason to have a child, but the way Fred treated me made me feel so useless and unloved. I needed love and my children were the source of that love. The doctor made me stay in bed for two weeks. My parents lived a few miles from us and helped with Tonya and Fred. My husband was a lot like another child, helpless around the house and with Tonya.

On and off, for the rest of the pregnancy, I had to be in bed. This angered my husband who wanted me to wait on him. Thank God, I had a healthy baby boy on July 11, 1973. This seemed to improve Fred's mood for a while, but then he decided he wanted to move his business to Florida. On top of that, I ruptured a disk in my back when my son was only three months old. This forced me into the hospital and I was in traction for two weeks. Even after I was released from the hospital they restricted me to bed. Again the two angels of mercy, my parents, stepped in to help us.

After the back injury, I remained depressed for a long time. I wanted to hold my new son and could not. I could hear my mother rocking him to sleep in the next room, and I have to admit I was jealous. I knew that was wrong, but I could not help myself. I should have been the one rocking him to sleep. The hurt and anger remained pent up in me like a tiger in a cage. My sadness lingered for many days and nights during that terrible time. I was so glad Mom was there to care for the children but hated that I could not do it myself. All I could think was that I was a terrible mother, not how lucky I was to have Mom there to help.

During this time my parents decided to move to Florida because of my father's ill health. Fred also wanted to relocate there. I really did not want to leave because all my friends were in Maryland but I decided that I could handle the move as long as my parents would be in Florida, too. I finally relented as usual to try to keep Fred happy.

After I began to recover, I found out that I was pregnant again. I guess it is surprising but once the doctor said I could have sex, my husband expected it right away. It took me seven years to get pregnant with my middle child and this one, a few months. Since I already had back problems my doctor required that I wear a back brace during the entire pregnancy. I had to be extremely careful when lifting my other my eight-month-old son but the brace really helped. The pain did not matter. The thought of having another child made me very happy and it took my mind off the sadness I had in my marriage. I had learned how to put on a happy face no matter what I felt. I was the proverbial crying clown.

My parents were in the process of buying a house in Florida. Mom had to continue working until the end of September to be eligible for full retirement. She stayed with Dad in Florida a few weeks to help him settle into their new home, but when her two weeks were up she had to return to Maryland for several months. Fred moved his business and left me behind to sell the house, pack up, and move everything to Florida. I felt so alone and abandoned. I had never done anything like that in my life. Here I was with a small baby and a seven-year-old daughter, and I was five months' pregnant. Many nights I cried myself to sleep with back pain and fear.

Except for occasional back pain, this pregnancy went very well. I did not spot at all and was able to get the house sold quickly. The only problem was the man who bought it wanted us out in a week. I did fight for an additional week and got it. I had started to pack but was not even close to being ready to get out. I look back and wonder how I did every-thing required of me without ending up in the hospital. God must have been watching over me. I packed everything up and we were on our way to Florida.

Then my father's illness worsened. It was one thing after another that year. He had a heart attack while sitting in the back seat of the car. We had been coming home from a birthday celebration. My mother and father both had birthdays within the same week. We were talking and laughing when he suddenly slumped over as if he fell asleep. At first my mother thought he was kidding around but then quickly realized something was wrong. We had just turned the corner and were a few blocks from our house. I knew he was having a heart attack since a year before he had a triple bypass and valve replacement surgery. Without thinking, I jumped over the seat and laid him down and started mouth-to-mouth resuscitation on him. When we pulled into the driveway of our home, I asked my husband to help me carry my father onto the lawn and my mother called the ambulance. I did my best to keep him alive. I had learned first aid as a Scout Leader but had never actually needed to use it on a real person. Now I tried with everything I had in me to do it correctly. This was my father. He and I had always understood each other. We were so much alike and so close. I had to bring him back to me. I just had to.

It seemed like hours until the ambulance arrived. I can remember everything, but it was all like a dream or an out-of-body experience. I remember seeing my mother, her hands shaking and looking drained. Dad's illness had taken a toll on her, now this. I was so grateful when the paramedics took over.

When we arrived at the hospital, he was still alive, but they said that he may have been without oxygen for too long. Despite my efforts, I may not have done everything necessary to save him. All I could hear or think was that I might have contributed to him living but with brain damage. Could I live with that?

I knew my father did not want to be kept alive by machines. Before his heart surgery, he talked to me about that exact thing. He did not want to upset my mother with such talk, but he knew I could take it. I was tough like him, or so he thought. I remember one day he looked at me and held my shoulders with his hands. "Don't ever let them put me on machines to keep me alive. Promise me?" I made that promise to him.

For my mother's sake, I knew that I had to be strong. All my feelings went into a deep place inside of me for the long haul.

My father lived on a respirator for one month. They knew he had brain damage but did not know the extent of it. While he remained in the intensive care unit, he could only have one visitor for five minutes once an hour. My mother, brother and I took turns going in to sit by him. Most of the time his eyes were closed, but one day I went in and he was looking at me. I felt daggers going though me. I reached out to hold his hand. He grabbed my hand and his eyes penetrated my soul. I just knew what he wanted to say to me. "You promised you would not let them do this to me." My brain logically told me that I did all I could, but then an avalanche of guilt fell upon me. Before I left the room, I had to get myself together for my mother. I just had to. Again I pushed my feelings below the surface to linger for many years. What I felt deep inside was that I had let my father down. I could barely look at myself in the mirror. I hated myself for trying to save him, for not letting him go. It was not my choice to make, but I could not help the way I felt. If I had not given him CPR, he would have died the way he wanted. I felt responsible.

He died a month after his heart attack. We lived in Florida, but being a veteran of the Air Force, he had a burial plot in Virginia, at Arlington Cemetery. My mother and brother took the first flight they could get to Washington, D.C. and my husband, children and I went by train the next day. It was a torturous trip and I do not remember much of it. I do recall being unable to sit with my children. I wanted to be with them in case they needed me but for some reason people did not want to move.

After a few incidents with the children, some disgusted man changed seats so I could complete the trip with my children at my side. I wondered what had taken him so long to figure that out. It is still a blur to this day.

The military funeral touched us all. The guilt of his final days weighed as heavy on me as the casket on the backs of the soldiers.

The train trip home was a nightmare. The bottom part of one of the cars, near the back of the train, caught on fire. We made about six stops to have fire engines put water on the car to keep it from starting again. One porter told us they did not have an area to drop the burning car so they had to make sure it did not spread. A normal nine-hour trip took us twenty-one hours.

Life changed for all of us forever. Dad's death started a downward spiral. We had to either sink or learn how to swim in order to get our lives back together.

*   *   *

That bout with the flu and my stress level had made me feel as if my nerves were right on the surface of my skin. During the days following my illness I had more trouble coping with my mother. I could not wait to return to work; I hated being home these days. At least work kept me busy so I could get my mind off what was happening at home. It seemed my life was always in turmoil. As soon as one thing went right, something else fell apart.

Work had always helped me feel like a determined, strong woman I had worked so hard to become. Now it was all I could do to get up in the morning. My energy level had decreased so much I barely had the strength to deal with my staff's problems perhaps because my own problems seemed insurmountable. What was happening to me? My brain did not seem to let me do my work. I kept wondering why I could not pull myself out of these doldrums as I always had in the past.

CHAPTER 3

January 20, 1993 I found myself dreading the tasks that were due by the end of the month. I never minded them before, as a matter of fact, I had enjoyed the challenge of completing everything in a timely manner. Not this year. Everything seemed different. The four employee reviews that were due, along with my yearly goals and my own review seemed to be at the top of a high mountain that I did not have the energy to climb. My brain seemed on autopilot. As I wrote the last paragraph on one of the reviews, I could not help thinking how stressful the last year and a half had been. I did not want to think about what 1993 would bring. I put the review in an envelope and walked over to the conference room where I was just in time for a meeting.

These days I did not enjoy the activities at work. I just vegetated while others talked. No longer did I give input or really care about what was said. About halfway through the meeting, a secretary called me out to take a phone call from Neighborhood House. Mom had lost control of her bladder. Normally I saw to it that she wore Depends undergarments in case she went for a walk, but this day Joe took her to day care and forgot to ask if she put one on. Since she had just started day care, I did not think to have a change of clothes there for her.

I called Joe, who offered to drive over to pick her up and take her home. My emotions were so close to the surface, but I knew I must never let myself be seen upset at work. All I could think of was my mother during that entire meeting. Should I have gone to get her? These meetings had become very important because they involved the reorganization of our areas. If they had not involved my staff, I would have left.

As I drove home, all that went through my mind was what might happen to my poor mother next. She still had very good bladder control most of the time. The only time she had a problem was if she went walking or had a cold. Occasionally I found wet underwear in one of her shoes or smell urine in her closet or room. When she was at day care, I followed the urine smell to find those dirty clothes and wash them, then clean and disinfect her room. We also kept a lined diaper pail in her bathroom so she could dispose of her Depends. She did not mind wearing them but often forgot to put them on unless Joe or I reminded her.

On the drive home from work, I tried to relax. I turned on an oldie's radio station. The music took me back to the seventies again. As I glanced out the window, I saw first graders walking alone the sidewalk. It reminded me of when my daughter was young.

*   *   *

Like her mother before her, Mom was always there when others needed her. She was very unselfish about that. She adored my children from the day they were born. Mom and Dad had enjoyed seven years with Tonya, my daughter, before my son Josh was born, so she had a special place in their hearts. Tonya loved helping my mother around the house and in the garden. Mom and Dad loved to travel and they often took Tonya on trips with them to see other relatives and to tour the U.S.

Mom had a real talent for decorating. Colors and fabrics seemed to fit together perfectly for her. She also excelled as a gardener. What a green thumb she had. She planted a seed and the most magnificent bush or flower grew in no time. Unfortunately, I did not receive any of those talents from her. I bought a new sofa for the house, brought it home, and it was either too large for the room or the color did not go with the curtains. It also seemed like I had a brown thumb; everything I planted turned brown within days.

Mom had been a tailor for years, during her hard times. When my daughter Tonya was small, my mother could sew a dress or coat for her in a few hours, and they looked better than anything in the stores. Since Mom never had much to call her own as a young person, she loved beautiful clothes and shoes. Not only did she enjoy buying them for herself, but she bought me lovely clothes and shoes when I was young, too. Then when Tonya came along, it was her turn. There again I was a disappointment to her. I could not sew worth a darn and never had the patience for it.

Mom always looked attractive even when she was working around the house. She loved a pretty hairstyle, and because I was a hairdresser back then, I often did her hair for her. I even treated her to facials and did her nails. I could tell it made her feel really pampered and relaxed, and it boosted her self-image.

She and my father had always been active and enjoyed life. They loved to go to parties, Knights of Columbus functions, plays, and out to dinner, and they really loved to travel. They even took a month long vacation overseas.

When Dad began having problems with his health, I could see it was affecting her, too. She was losing part of herself as his illness became worse. Her eyes grew swollen and dark circles formed from her lack of sleep. She seemed to be in a daze most of the time. I think now that she must have been feeling shock. She just could not imagine life without the man who had become a part of her.

A short time after my father died, my divorce was finalized. Fred became even more abusive as his business failed. He drank all the time. Oh, he did not beat us or anything that bad, but he was cruel and lost his temper. He scared the daylights out of all of us. I remember the time he got mad because his beer did not fit in the refrigerator. He pulled out a watermelon, took it to the driveway, and threw it down hard, breaking it open. It reminded me of a head. I know that sounds terrible, but it frightened me. He did the same thing with Venetian blinds once. He tried putting them up, had problems doing it, and just threw them into the outside garbage can. These incidents made me realize how violent he could be over nothing. I worried about the children.

The night Fred carried my son by the neck to his bedroom, I knew I had to get the man out of our lives. He could mentally abuse me but when he started to physically abuse the children, I could not put up with that. I had enough and I told him I wanted him out. He just laughed and said, "What the hell do you think you can do? You will be crawling back to me to support you and the kids in two days." He was wrong. My years of torment and mental abuse from this man had ended. I did not care what I had to do.

Times were about to get worse. I had to begin to build a life for the children and me. My salary did not cover the bills. At one point, my husband wanted me to take him back. During that weak point, I had him to sign a Quick Claim Deed to put the house in my name. I told him he should want the children to have a roof over their heads no matter what happened between us. I still cannot believe I had the courage to do it or that he agreed. Now my only worry was making the monthly house payments.

Stress began to increase. I had so many things to do and became desperate to find a sitter for my children while I worked. Day care cost more than I made at my job, and none of them were open at nights when I worked. Since my mother hated living alone, and I needed a babysitter, she offered to move in with me. She knew that she would have to give up some of her favorite activities like playing bridge, bowling and church work. All of those activities took place in the evenings and that is when she would be babysitting.

She had taught me well, though. I knew a woman could make it. I had both my mother and grandmother as role models and three excellent reasons to try. I worried I could never be as good at anything as my mother. Now I wished I had gone to college. I kept thinking that if I worked hard enough at my job, I would succeed. I knew it was going to be difficult, but I could do it.

All the women in my family, from as far back as my great-grandmother, passed down good work ethics to my brother and me. My mother had worked for the government for many years before her retirement. She took care of the family finances and paperwork. She was well known for her meticulous, well-organized clerical abilities. I have to admit she was not the world's greatest housekeeper. Once I had to work outside the home and be a mother and wife, I understood why.

Mom had worked in Washington, D.C., as an executive secretary for many years. During that time, she had many younger friends. She enjoyed life and felt young, so she fit right in with a more youthful group. They often lunched and went out shopping and to see the wonderful sights in Washington, D.C. On the weekends, she went golfing, bowling, or played bridge with her friends. Mom kept up with the younger crowd, and they just loved her company. They often told me how great she was.

She had an interesting work life. I remember her sitting at the dinner table one night talking about the day a high-ranking government official involved in the Watergate scandal, hid in the office down the hall from her to avoid the press. We used to tease her about being the paper shredder during the Watergate scandal and asked her what she did with the tapes. At the time, most of what she knew had to be kept secret. She had knowledge of a great deal of top-secret government material. We knew better than to ask her about any of it. She held her job and her responsibilities' sacred.

Having a mother who seemed so perfect in my mind made it difficult for me. No matter how I tried, I could not help worrying. My failures could disappoint my children and my mother yet again. I often wondered if I could ever live up to what others expected of me. No matter how hard I tried, I always seemed to mess things up.

CHAPTER 4

I finally had a day off. The weather was exceptionally warm for the first of February. Mom and I were both tired of being inside. We had enough of the cold and snow that the winter of 1993 had dumped on us. Every day possible, I took her outside for a walk, even if it was just around the church property across the street.

I was so tired these days from lack of sleep. Maybe I could get Mom to relax outside and give me some rest. I set up two lawn chairs out in the back yard and put the radio on the picnic table. After turning the radio on, I looked out over the pastureland behind our home and could see nothing but high weeds dried up from the winter cold. The little red barn that had always been the landmark to our house was deserted now. I watched the neighbors' horses and sheep munch on grass in their pastures and thought of so many wonderful times when our yard was filled with laughing children and happy adults. So much had changed. All of the children who once played there were grown, and the only sound left was trees rustling in the wind. On top of that emptiness, I felt like I was losing Mom a little more each day.

I brought some houseplants out to the picnic table to repot. Mom loved being outside. She had a little spring in her step as she helped me by carrying some gardening tools to the back yard. Our cat followed us, nearly tripping me as I came down the porch stoop. As soon as my mother got to the picnic table, she put down the tools and picked up the cat who had curled her tail around Mom's leg and meowed. The cat loved the attention and my mother seemed to be enjoying herself.

A slight breeze kept the air chilly, but it was warm enough to enjoy being outside. I began to open bags of potting soil to put some dirt into the new pots. Mom watched while she petted the cat. I felt more like going to sleep on one of the lawn chairs but knew Mom might take off down the street if I did.

As I placed a plant into new soil, my mind could not stop racing. I kept trying to figure out a way to attend some of the Alzheimer's support group sessions. I had tried fitting it into my work schedule but the times never worked out, and I was too exhausted to add anything else to my already hectic days. I needed to be with others in the same situation, but in a way I felt like family illnesses should be kept private. If I were to share my fears with strangers, no matter how understanding they were, I felt it was a sign of weakness. I knew I owed it to Mom to find a way to do this, but I could find no solution.

The cat was playing with the new bracelet on Mom's wrist. A simple thing like this bracelet took such a worry off my mind. For months, Mom snuck out of the house and walked down the road. We constantly worried about her running off and not remembering where she lived. I had a brainstorm one day after just such an incident and asked Joe if we could have a special identification bracelet made for her. We bought a gold identification bracelet and had it engraved with her name and phone number on one side and our address on the other.

The cat sat curled up on Mom's lap, but Mom was no longer petting her. Her arms were down at her sides. She looked as if she did not even realize the cat was still sitting there. She was mentally somewhere else these days. She became very agitated or she sat with a blank stare. I had to fight the tears away when I saw her get that way. Only a few years ago, she could never relax without a book to read. She never watched TV except for her taped "soap operas."

I went over to her and held her hand for a minute. "Come on, Mom, I need your help. You know me. I'm the one with the brown thumb in the family. Your touch makes things grow."

It took a minute, but Mom seemed to snap out of it and slowly got up. I led her over to the picnic table and put a dirt scoop into her hand. She always liked being right beside me no matter what I was doing. She used to love gardening, but these days I wondered if she had any idea what I was doing.

As I looked at the beautiful plants, I felt guilty for how much I hated God these days. I had such a difficult time understanding why God did this terrible thing to such a wonderful woman. Every Sunday I took her to church where she gazed at the back of the person in front of her. At times, she seemed to have no idea why she was there. Mom had always been a very religious person. She came from a family of devout Catholics. Several times in my life, I left the fold and this was one of those times. I knew I may disappoint Mom yet again, but I could not help turning my anger and resentment toward a God who could hurt my mother.

When we finished, I cleaned up both of us and put our newly potted plants back in the house. I had been right to let Mom get some fresh air. She was not in the house but a few minutes when I noticed her dozing off in her favorite rocking chair. I started dinner while she slept. Again my mind drifted to the past.

*   *   *

After my divorce in 1977, I had to work two and sometimes three jobs just to make ends meet. Fred lived up to his threat. Right after the divorce was final, he took off and left us financially devastated. He never sent a penny of the child support he owed. Because he was self-employed the courts were unable to trace him. My parents had raised me to take care of myself and not to depend upon others. So I worked, and worked and worked. The most stressful thing was answering nasty phone calls dealing with my ex-husband's creditors. It was bad enough that I had to pay off the credit we owed personally, but his business creditors called constantly, as did the I.R.S.

During that time, Mom worked as an executive secretary for a government agency. We took turns watching and caring for the children. I felt so bad when the children asked for grandma and did not listen to me. But Mom was with them both mentally and physically, and I was not. I still had so much anxiety and anger about the divorce and Fred taking off, that I did not seem to be able to relate to the children well during that time period. Again, I needed to keep my feelings in check because Mom was still recovering from my father's death. Being with the children gave her new purpose. The children kept both of us busy. Despite our differences, I could see the parallel between my mother and me during this time. We both threw ourselves into our work to try to get past the sorrow, and to avoid the fear of what may be ahead.

Having my mother there with the children gave them a strong emotional support. She read to them, played games with them, kept them fed and clean, and loved them. I knew that they may not turn out to be strong adults without her wonderful care and love. I also think they helped her. She always gave my father so much love, and now she needed an outlet for that love. The children were fortunate enough to be that outlet.

There were good times, too. I remember one really funny incident in particular when we lived in South Florida. Because I worked night shift, every Saturday Mom watched the children so that I could sleep until noon. One Saturday Mom came in, woke me from a sound sleep and told me I had to come with her. I followed in a daze. My eyes were barely open and I had not fully awakened yet. She pushed me onto the porch. "It's a snake. Kill it!" She said, and then she slammed the sliding door behind me locking it. There I stood, in my robe, looking at this five-foot snake of some kind. The snake seemed to look back at me. I am not sure who was more scared. I can say it woke me up fast. Slowly and quietly, I turned to the door and said to Mom, "Get me a hoe or a shovel." She ran to the garage and brought back a garden hoe. She opened the door just enough to get the hoe through it, then slammed it again. Maybe the vibration of the slamming door made the snake decide it was not that thrilled being there. It went back outside through a hole in the screened-in porch. I chased after it until it slithered into a drainpipe on the other side of the fence. Naturally, I did not go back to sleep that day. Afterward, the children, Mom and I had a good laugh about it. I asked her if she thought I was going to kill it with my bare hands. She said, "Sure." After that incident, Mom and I had a deal. She killed the bugs, and I killed the snakes. It worked out well for both of us because I hated bugs. I especially dreaded hearing the shells on those palmetto bugs crunch, but Mom picked them up in a tissue and squeezed them until they popped.

In order to advance at my primary job, I decided to return to college. Most of the students were there right out of high school. That intimidated me since I had been out of school for fifteen years. If I could expand my knowledge of computers, I could apply to a higher-paying job in that area and give up some of those extra jobs. Many days, I went to work on four to five hours of sleep. It seemed to be enough. I carried so much guilt, frustration, and anger with me that I did not sleep well anyway.

About six months from the time Fred and I were divorced, life started to calm down. I received a promotion that gave me the money I needed to quit my second job. I had a better outlook and felt proud that I had accomplished so much on my own. The time I spent with my children became fun for me, and they loved it. Mostly I wanted to be their mother again.

Often I thought it was a good thing that Mom and I worked different parts of the day. We did not have to be around each other, and I could avoid arguments about our different philosophies on how to raise the children. Our relationship had always been a little tense, but it was even worse now. I knew I loved my mother, but I hated the way she attempted to raise my children when I was not home. I began to realize that some of the problems that caused me to have low self-esteem were being repeated in my children. She taught me to believe that what I did was not my best. I needed to work harder, be stronger, be prettier. She never wanted her children to have "swelled heads" and felt that pointing out our deficiencies was better than building our confidence. Just as she had pointed out my faults, she was now doing the same with my children. I hated to say anything because I did not want to start an argument. After all, I did not want to seem ungrateful to her.

Mom worried about everything her entire life. During my teen years, we tried our best to get along but we were so different. It was tough for both of us, but we had a lot of fun and had enjoyable times, too. I remember one year on her birthday, the children and I bought her a tee shirt with the saying, "Don't Worry, Be Happy." Anything involving the children gave us reason to get along, and our love for them overflowed into our relationship.

Later in my life, I figured out that her negativity came from her life. She was afraid to think anything good could happen. During the Depression, responsibilities took priority over one's dreams. She had always been an excellent student and even received a full scholarship to college. Mom had to help her mother raise her brothers and sister so she had to work instead of accepting the scholarship. I know that had to have had a tremendous impact upon her attitude about life.

For several years after the divorce, survival came from working as a team. Eventually, my mother, the children and I grew closer. We had more time for fun activities. I realized later that I had simply learned how to push my feelings below the surface in order to avoid confrontation. This became a normal part of life for me. I taught myself how to keep my feelings inside and never let them show, except for love.

*   *   *

As I watched my mother sleeping peacefully in her rocking chair, I became aware that we had always loved each other but we did not always like each other. Now, all I could feel was sadness and regret for all the time we had spent being angry with each other. I wished that I had attempted to understand her better when she was still well. Unfortunately, that lost time could never be regained, and any chance to make up for it was gone.

CHAPTER 5

The second Sunday in February 1993, Joe and I sat at the dining room table reading the newspaper. Mom came out of her room looking confused.

She held a picture up to me and asked, "Who is this?"

As I took the picture from her, I felt the blood drain from my face. "This was your husband, John, Mom. My father. You were married to him for more than forty years."

"So I know this person?" she asked, still not understanding what I had said.

"Yes, you loved him very much." I had to get up and go into the bedroom. Joe took over talking to her. He knew this was too much for me. My composure was cracking and he knew I did not want to upset her. I took the picture of my father into the bedroom. Through my tears I remembered how difficult it was after he died and my divorce became final.

*   *   *

The late seventies and early eighties had meant struggles for all of us. Mom and I had successfully maintained the house payments, fed and clothed the children. We made our meals stretch by using Mom's old recipes that she and her mother used during the Depression. Our meals were fixed with noodles, potatoes or rice mixed in with vegetables or meat. This helped to expand the meals so we had enough to feed all of us. We still made sure the children had their greens and fruits. We cut ads from the paper, magazines and newspapers and bought an occasional turkey or roast. The children learned to enjoy our creative dishes.

After three years of working, going to school, and learning to live as a single mother, I met Joe. The children and my mother liked him right away. Mom encouraged the relationship. She often made special dinners and invited him whenever we both had time off, which was not very often. Joe and his friends were wonderful with the children. They would laugh, play games and just be there for them. Mom told me that she thought they needed a positive male role model and I agreed.

We dated for a year. I worked nights and Joe worked days so we had limited time together. I guess I was a little old-fashioned, but I never let him sleep at our house. When he proposed marriage, I hesitated. Joe had never been married before, and I did not know how he would handle being a full-time father of three. My children came first. I also could not ask my mother to leave after all she had done for my children and me.

After two years of dating, I agreed to accept his marriage proposal. Joe insisted that everything stay the same. He asked that my mother continue to live with us, and he promised to raise the children as his own. I was nervous after my failed marriage, but we were in love and it felt right. Joe differed from Fred in so many ways. He was the most honest person I had ever met. If he said something, I knew I could count on it to be true.

That was a very happy time in our home. The wedding preparations brought us all close together. My happiness spilled over to my mother and the children. One of my fondest memories is shopping for my wedding dress with my mother and daughter. I had been married before but never had a big wedding. This time I wanted to look special. I tried on dress after dress and we laughed and had fun the entire day.

Mom took great pleasure in being involved in the events and made sure things were on track in her usual organized way. I wore a long ivory dress with a spring hat. My two sons, Josh and Matt, were ring bearers and my daughter Tonya was the maid of honor. My brother walked me down the isle. Mom made Tonya's dress and the two ring bearer pillows. Joe's family came, and the entire day was a dream. During the beginning of the ceremony, Joe and I each carried a rose to our mothers to show them how special they were to us.

We had a wonderful marriage, but like all marriages, we had our rough times, too. Being the youngest in his family, Joe had never been around many children. He expected our children to act more grown up than they were. We talked things out and eventually we both grew to be better parents. My mother and I had always been a bit too lenient with the children and Joe now gave them the balance they needed. The children loved and respected him, and Joe got along better with my mother than I did. She respected him and knew he wanted to do right by the family.

Joe came from a strong Italian background and family was very important to him. His mother and father were wonderful to all of us. I had heard horror stories from friends who had remarried after a divorce. Often the in-laws made life miserable for them and their children. This was never the case with Joe's parents. I thought since Joe had never been married, his parents might resist a marriage to a woman with a ready-made family. That was not the case at all. They accepted all of us without hesitation. His parents, Elizabeth and Salvador treated us like we had always been a part of their family. Mom fit in very well. They were around the same age and always had a lot to talk about. Mom rarely played cards at home but during our times with Joe's parents the evening ended with coffee, dessert and playing card games. Elizabeth and Salvador opened their home and their hearts to us all.

Not long after our marriage, Joe asked the children and me if he could adopt them. It was not a difficult thing because their father had abandoned them. Since we were unable to find Fred, the courts required permission for their adoption from Fred's mother. She agreed and signed the necessary papers. Joe's wish to make the children part of a whole family became reality. My mother stood proudly as she watched the judge preside over the adoption. Afterward we went out to dinner to celebrate. Mom told me later that I could not have chosen a better man to raise my children. I agreed.

That same year, Joe's company wanted him to move from Florida to Utah. The entire family discussed the move and everyone agreed to it. Joe made certain my mother understood this also meant her. To our surprise Mom loved the idea. The children agreed although Tonya was a bit reluctant to move away and start a new high school. She did, however, love horses and the west seemed to be very appealing to her. After considerable discussion, we all agreed that living out west might be the perfect start for our new marriage and family.

We were adjusting to being a family, and this move was yet another challenge. Josh and Matt were small enough that they did not really have a problem moving. Since Mom and I had lived a military life for so many years, we were used to packing up and moving at a moment's notice.

The closer we got to the move, the more excited my mother became. She told me she could not wait to begin our new adventure. I laughed and told her she just missed all that moving she used to do in the Air Force. She agreed and said it had always been something she enjoyed. In Florida, we had lived in a small home on a corner lot but now we had an acre of land with a large ranch style home on it. Each child had his or her own room, and my mother had her own bedroom and bathroom. We even had a little red barn, a pasture, and two horses.

I worked for the same company as Joe, so before we moved I had a contract for a job at the new location. I started working within a few weeks of moving into the house. Joe and I had technical jobs that required us to work odd shifts, and we had to be on call at times. Since

Mom had her own transportation, it did not take her long to find a job herself. While the children were in school, she worked at the church doing office work. She enjoyed working with the priest and nuns and began to socialize with her church group. She joined a bowling league and often lunched and took day trips with her friends. We quickly settled into our new surroundings.

Moving to Utah and the country became a learning experience for us all. Not only had none of us ever lived in the country before but we were now the minority in a nearly all-Mormon neighborhood. Our Air Force experiences had taught us how to live among people who had different beliefs and interests. Our neighbors were great and helped us figure out what we needed to do to take care of our mini farm.

We enjoyed the strict Mormon lifestyles. They did not drink and abstained from using drugs. They were family-oriented and many women still stayed at home with their children. I was the only woman on my block working outside the home. We were shocked at how large the families were in Utah. In Florida, I was considered to have a large family with three children. Many families in Utah had from seven to twelve children. Our differences, however, did not prevent us from living happily among them. My mother loved the neighbors and quickly became the neighborhood grandma. She had a way of making children feel right at home and very important. Her special homemade treats were always a hit with the children.

I joined the Boy Scout Committee at the neighborhood Latter-day Saints (L.D.S.) Ward. The Mormon Church supported most of the Scouts and sports. As the lone woman on the Committee, I filled in doing whatever type of help they needed. Once they asked me to type the Ward phone book (A Ward is the Mormon meeting place.) Since our family was not Mormon, we were not going to be in it. We all made a real breakthrough for diversity during that discussion in deciding to call the book our Neighborhood Phone Book instead of the Ward

Phone book. They decided to put the names of all neighbors, despite their religious beliefs, in the book. We learned a lot from each other.

Josh and Matt joined Little League Baseball and the Scouts, and before long they fit right in with the neighbors. Tonya joined Future Farmers of America and made friends in the cowboys' circuit. Joe and I both worked full-time. Mom loved her secretarial work for the church and became very active in golf, bowling, and socializing in general.

We city slickers found living in the country very interesting. I remember the day Joe and I came home from work to find my mother laughing. She said, "You will not believe what happened to me today."

"What?" I asked.

"I heard the doorbell this morning and went to the door to find two police officers standing there. The officer asked me if I knew our sheep were out. I said we did not own any sheep. He said, 'You do now.' The officer moved out of my way and I saw sheep covering our entire front yard, grazing on our grass and flowers." Our neighbor's sheep had broken through their fence and I guess our grass looked good to them. The police proceeded to let the neighbor know and soon Mom watched her first round-up from the front door.

Another funny thing that happened related to my daughter. Tonya raised a sheep for a project for Future Farmers of America. That baby lamb kept us awake the entire first week. The fence Joe built for the lamb was right outside our bedroom window. Like all baby animals, it cried for a while when taken away from its mother. Having been born and raised in New York City, Joe found it strange to have animal sounds, instead of traffic sounds, keeping him awake.

Mom decided that learning about growing vegetables in a garden might be a good learning experience for the children. She and Joe tilled and prepared the garden. We all planted, and enjoyed watching the vegetables begin to bud. The children helped her pull weeds and pick the vegetables when the time was right. Although I never had her green thumb, she even got me involved by showing me how to blanch and freeze the vegetables for later use. I also learned to cook zucchini a thousand ways, since we had planted way too many seedlings. The children loved zucchini bread and cookies; Joe, Mom and I loved the baked zucchini. I nearly spent my entire food budget on nuts and flour that year. Because Joe and I worked so many hours, Mom taught our children how to grow food, a life lesson that they may not otherwise have learned.

During summer of 1983, floods hit Utah. It was the year that they built a wall of sandbags that lined one of the main city streets. This enabled the water from mountain runoff to flow down the creeks and into the street, making it a river of downtown Salt Lake City. Our street was no exception. The basement, which we had finished just before we moved into the house, flooded. High ground water backed up our septic tanks. The entire neighborhood chipped in to help each other by sharing sump pumps and water vacuums, and our co-workers brought us some pallets to put our furniture on. Most of the time we were so busy we did not have time to think about the damage. It all hit me as I stood watching the Disaster Cleanup company carry my brand-new, not-yet-paid-for carpet from the basement. As they carried that dripping carpet out the door, Mom said, "Just think what we have been through in our lives. At least we are all healthy and no one was hurt. These are things. Things can be replaced. Your family can't."

We checked around to find out what could be done about the high-water-table problem during flood years. Finally we decided to have someone put in French Drains. This meant digging a moat below the foundation of our house. We were ready to find any method that would help us fix the problem.

During this entire time, about three months, we had to use a porta potty and bury our waist. Since water use had to be limited, we could only use minimal water for showering, doing dishes, and cooking. We felt like pioneers. I was so grateful to have my mother there during that time. She brought humor into the situation. Each day she took the children and went to the library, a store, or out for a snack. The actual purpose was to use a real bathroom. The neighbors were in the same situation so we could not ask them for help.

Mom's life during the Depression and the difficulty of helping her mother, brothers and sister during that time, taught her how to survive. Now she shared what she learned with us. For example, one day during our high-water problems, Tonya wanted to be able to wash her long hair. My mother came up with the idea to run a hose from the kitchen window to the yard so Tonya could get a good hair-washing. The water was even warm. Once again, Mom had come through for us.

We had years of ups and downs, but overall we did manage. In 1985, Tonya went away to Southern Utah University. My mother and I had a great time attending to both of my boys' basketball games and different functions at their school. We both cheered and clapped until our hands were sore. Mom loved it when the boys brought all their friends to the house and ate everything in sight. She and I were as close as we had ever been. We shopped and had ladies' time out together. Because I worked a three-and-a-half-day week, I had a lot of time off during the weekdays.

Once Tonya graduated from college in 1989 and went to live and work about an hour's drive from our home, things began to change. We no longer had horses. Josh left for college, and Matt was a normal high-school student about to graduate. Just before Josh left for college, the three children, Joe and I made one last trip together.

In September of 1990, Joe's parents celebrated their 50th wedding anniversary. We planned for my mother to fly to St. Louis to stay with her brother while we drove with the family to Florida. We stopped at Disney World for three days, then drove to South Florida. The anniversary party went perfectly. Everyone was happy and the occasion could not have been better. Elizabeth and Salvador made the perfect couple. Everyone danced, ate, and enjoyed each other's company. Wonderful memories were made for everyone that day.

Just before we left, we received a call from my uncle. My mother had been out for a walk with him and passed out. They took her to the hospital and ran some tests. Twenty years before, she had her thyroid removed and had been on medication every day since. Evidently the medication suddenly became ineffective and caused her to faint. They had to readjust her medication. We asked my uncle if she wanted to fly home or if we should stop by and pick her up on our way back. He said she wanted to return home with us. We left Florida a day early and arrived in St. Louis two days later. Her appearance surprised me. She looked especially weak and pale. I could not wait to get her home, but I knew the trip was not going to be easy for her.

Once we arrived home, I could tell my mother was not herself. We had to take her to the hospital a few times. The doctor had her on medication to regulate her irregular heartbeat that appeared to cause her the most problems. He had us check her pulse throughout the day to make sure she was doing all right. She seemed lethargic and still had no energy.

I became concerned and went out to buy a book on side effects and interaction of medications and began to monitor my mother's symptoms. The next time I took her to the doctor I discussed what I had found out, and read him the notes I had taken. I made certain to discuss this with him in private and did not want to make Mom feel bad. She had so much pride. I had never tried to talk to a doctor like that before. It was an uncomfortable feeling. As I read the notes to the doctor, I told him that I was not trying to tell him what to do. I was with her every day and did not think she was doing well.

He accepted my opinion and went on to explain what they had been doing. He agreed we could cut out at least one medication as long as I monitored her reaction. I promised to take good care of her. Joe, Matt and I took turns monitoring her and taking her pulse. She seemed much less lethargic and her memory seemed better for a few weeks. I was so relieved and thought the worst was behind us.

＊   ＊   ＊

As I put the picture of my father in the album, I looked at some other pictures. Did Mom remember our wedding, the move to Utah or anything else? Did she know any of her family? I could not help thinking that she may not even know me at times. How sad that a person fills a life with so much, as she did, and then loses it all at the end. I always thought that if nothing else, we always had our memories. Now I was not so sure.

CHAPTER 6

The third week of February 1993, Mom put a spoon in the microwave. Luckily I caught the problem before she hit the start button. Later that day I looked in Mom's closet for dirty clothes to wash. I found clothes stuffed in one of her shoes. On occasion I came across other items like her watch in the refrigerator and her purse in the bathtub. These days she misplaced her belongings often. The most difficult to find were her false teeth. Once I found them wrapped in a tissue in a box in her closet. It happened so frequently that I began to know the places she would often hide things.

After I put the laundry in the washer, we went to the foot doctor and grocery store. I remembered how astute she had always been when it came to shopping. Now she just walked along with me like a small child with no concept of why we were there. That night I asked her if she wanted to help me make dinner. She said, "Make what?" It may not sound like much, but after years of doing all the cooking, now my mother did not know what dinner was. I hated how this disease was stealing my mother's memories.

*   *   *

After the visit with her brother in 1990, I began to notice Mom seemed different. The problems resulting from her thyroid medication not only hospitalized her but we began to notice subtle changes in her.

Over the fifteen years Mom lived with us, she would often do things that made her look helpless so others could cater to her. When her confusion started, both Joe and I thought she was just trying to get attention. It was a game she played, like when the lady of the manor fainted. We understood her and played along, usually giving in to her. We did not mind giving her what she wanted, but these times were occurring more often. Joe and I wondered if more could be going on than we had first thought.

The longer she acted this way, the clearer it became that something was not right. At first I tried to convince myself that it was just her age. Joe and I thought that she was just becoming more forgetful or that she had not recovered from her illness. The little things really bothered me. She had always been obsessive about her papers and money. Suddenly, she became almost secretive about her room and belongings.

A couple of years before her illness, she had shown me where to look for important information in case anything ever happened to her. Not a paper was out of place. She had organized and filed everything perfectly and had put either my brother Robert's or my name on all of her bank accounts and financial documents. Her brother, David, had convinced her to do that, and because he was very knowledgeable about finances, she always listened to him. After he had talked to her about what to do, she set up everything the way he suggested. Then she took me to the bank to add my name to her safe deposit box, gave me an extra key, and told me she had Certificates of Deposit in it.

Of course, I was shocked when she asked me to help her balance her checkbook. I was the one who usually needed her help with my check-book. Before she retired, she was the executive secretary for a member of the Cabinet in Washington, D.C. Her wide range of skills had always carried over to her personal papers and accounts, but now things were different.

When I started to work on her checkbook, I could not believe how her writing and entries had changed over the past few months. I also noticed that she had not added her direct deposits from Social Security and her pension into the check register, and she had not paid several of her bills that were due. Mom had always paid everything ahead of time but when I asked her about it, she said that they had slipped her mind. Many check entries were missing or incorrect. The status of her checkbook heightened my concern. This was not my mother; she had never let her checkbook get this bad.

Later that night, I talked to Joe about it. He said that she may still be suffering some memory loss from her illness and that she may improve with time. I agreed, but in the back of my mind I had a nagging feeling something was not right. If asked to put it into words, I would have said, "Mom is slowly losing her abilities." I made a note to ask her doctor why she seemed to be having these problems. She had just been to the doctor's office during the past week, so was not due for another appointment for two months. I decided I should probably not wait. I would make a call to the doctor and ask if the problems could be a side effect of her medication or illness. I hoped the doctor would be able to treat her and help her get back to the way she had once been.

Before I had a chance to call the doctor the next morning, we received a call that one of my uncles had died. Uncle David and my mother had always been very close, but Mom still was not well enough to travel from Utah to Pennsylvania, so my brother Robert and I decided to make the trip to the funeral. The loss of our uncle had a deep impact on my brother and me. Our father and mother had traveled and been best friends with Uncle David and his wife Aunt Grace for many years, and David's death brought back memories of our father.

I did not really like to travel alone, but I knew I had to go. My brother drove to Pennsylvania from Wisconsin. I flew in from Utah.

Until I was at the funeral, I was not aware of just how close to the surface my emotions were. I did not know what a toll my mother's illness had taken on me. I had been so busy, between work and driving her back and forth to the doctors, that I did not have time to think about myself. It was very strange to suddenly discover at the funeral that I could not keep up my normal facade. I had always done that very well, but not this time. After the service, I literally sobbed to the point of total embarrassment. I could not seem to stop myself.

Within two months of my Uncle David's death, my thirty-one-year-old cousin died of brain cancer. Then my mother's youngest brother died within three months of his brother David. I think all of these deaths so close together devastated my mother more than she let on. She kept her emotions inside, too. Apparently I learned that from her.

After returning from the funeral, I could never seem to get Mom off my mind. Every day at work had become more of a chore. I used to enjoy coaching my staff and working through new ideas, but now I could barely concentrate. My mind was on Mom.

I had always been actively involved in my work, and I rarely procrastinated. I used to drive my boss crazy because I would have work done within an hour after he gave it to me. He would say, "Don't do that, you are making me work too hard." We would both laugh and get back to work. These days I could barely think. I could no longer come up with solutions to problems presented by my staff. Making it through my day had now become as monumental to me as climbing the Empire State Building.

Although work was a great distraction, I found it difficult to keep up that happy front all the time. Looking back, I know I should have found someone to talk to, but I had always dealt with my problems by myself or with Joe's help. Now we were both in the same situation, and we were not much help to each other. I wish that I had swallowed my pride and gone to a psychologist or at least attended a support group.

After the staff meeting wrapped up, someone asked me if I was all right. Not wanting to go into a lengthy discussion about my personal life, I just said I was a little under the weather, my ongoing excuse for being preoccupied.

I rarely took a lunch hour, but this day I did. I needed to get out of the office, to drive around the city and try to relax. As I passed the bank where my mother had her accounts, I remembered her second incident concerning the bank.

When Mom returned home from a trip to the bank that day, she had the contents of her safe deposit box in a shopping bag. When I asked her why she had taken her things out of the bank, she said that she did not know. Her blank expression had worried me. It was a look I had seen more often as time had gone on.

Later that day, a bank clerk had called. She told me that she hated to let my mother remove the contents from her safe deposit box but did not really have a choice. She just wanted to make sure someone in the family was aware of her action. She also said that my mother had come in last week and was making no sense at all. "I tried to help her as much as I could. I asked her if she needed a balance on her account. Your mother didn't answer. She just turned around and left," she told me.

I had promised the clerk that I would accompany my mother to the bank in the future, and I thanked her for being so thoughtful. I appreciated living in a place where people seemed to care about others and did not fear being involved.

I could not hold back the tears as I passed the bank. My make-up ran down my face. I pulled into McDonald's restaurant near the bank to repair my make-up and buy lunch. I hated myself more every day, and I cried every time I was alone. I was becoming an out-of-control crybaby. My already overweight body seemed to crave the hamburger and fries I consumed. In the back of my mind, I kept thinking that maybe if I died of a heart attack, I could avoid being the next one in my family to suffer with the same disease that my mother had now.

* * *

I took Mom into the kitchen with me and got out the plates for her to set the table for dinner. I thought that I should keep her active. I felt sure that keeping busy would help her maintain mental, as well as her physical, health.

Mom looked confused when I handed her the plates. Once she got to the table, I noticed that she just stood there, not sure of what to do next. I went and stood beside her with my arm around her shoulders. "Let's see if we can do something different tonight. What if we put the plate here?" As I showed her where to place things, she followed behind me doing what I asked. I had to show her where each plate, knife, fork and spoons were supposed to go. I wondered how many times she had set a table in her life. Now she had to have my help for this simple task. Each day Mom seemed to be losing more of herself. Was there anything more that I could do to help her save herself?

CHAPTER 7

February 23, 1993 I had just returned to my office when Joe rushed in. "I just got another call from Neighborhood House about your Mom. One of us needs to go pick her up again." He looked tired. She seemed to be doing well at Neighborhood House and even enjoyed going there. There were times, though, when even that confused her.

"Is she all right? What happened?"

"For some reason, when the bus arrived to pick up some other seniors, she started to scream that they came to put her in jail. They cannot seem to calm her down. I'm just about to leave anyway, so I'll go get her. I hope she knows me. I don't know how I'm going to get her to come home with me if not," Joe said.

Joe knew that she had recently had lapses and did not know the family.

"Maybe I should take off and go with you."

"No, it's okay. I'll call you if I can't get her to calm down. Otherwise, I'll see you at home later."

"Are you sure?"

"Yes. She will probably be calmed down by the time I get there anyway."

We were both starting to worry that a few more incidents like this one and the Neighborhood House could not handle her. Neither of us talked about it, but we wondered what we would do then.

I returned to my desk but I could not concentrate. I looked at a picture I had of Mom and her brother Steven and thought back to when I had taken it.

*   *   *

In spring of 1992, Mom's brother Steven planned to spend his vacation by taking Mom to Las Vegas to visit relatives. When he arrived at our home, I was happy to see him but concerned about what was happening with my mother. I did the best I could to explain to him the strange state she was in. He said the trip would be a good change for her. I was not too sure about that. It seemed that any type of change these days seemed to confuse and upset her. In all honesty, however, it was a relief for her to go with Steven. Joe and I needed some time alone. In all the years we had been married, we had rarely been alone in the house, and had seldom even been alone together. Our nerves had been on edge for many months now, and I hoped we might actually get a full night's sleep while Mom was gone.

It was good to see that Mom recognized her brother. As they drove away, I felt like I did when I put my children on the bus for their first day of school. I knew how Mom had changed, but I was afraid that I had not given Steven enough information to keep her safe, especially in a place the size of Las Vegas.

Steven only called me once while they were on their trip. He said everything was fine but that Mom was constantly searching for her purse. That was one thing I had forgotten to warn him about, her misplacing her purse and her obsession with finding it. Steven was always able to find the purse in some strange place, like under her bed or behind a door.

When they returned home, Steven confirmed my warning to him that she was not able to adapt well to unfamiliar surroundings. The crowded casinos and all the noise from the slot machines made her very nervous. He also said that on the way home she thought some men in a nearby car were going to shoot at them. Now it seemed that, in addition to her confusion, Mom was becoming paranoid.

The day after Mom returned from her trip, I called her doctor and updated him on her condition, especially about the paranoia she experienced while on her trip with Steven. I told him about other incidents such as finding her important personal papers thrown in her trash can. I also explained about her driving problems. He told me to bring her in for a checkup.

When I told Mom that I was taking her to the doctor, she insisted, "I don't need to go to the doctor. I'm not sick." I finally convinced her to go. As we approached the office, Mom stopped in her tracks. I had to talk to her for quite a while before she finally went inside. When the nurse called her name, Mom argued with me and said she was leaving. Nothing I said or did could persuade her to go with the nurse. Mom was yelling that she did not want any man touching her as the other patients in the waiting room tried not to stare at her. The nurse asked the receptionist to get the doctor. When they came into the waiting room, the doctor sat on the sofa and calmly said he was happy to see her. She seemed to be taken off-guard by the change of tactics and stood motionless for a moment. I could only sit stunned while they patiently calmed my mother. After a considerable time of just chatting with Mom, the doctor and his nurse finally were able to reassure her, and she consented to the exam.

The doctor never mentioned anything to me about the notes I had taken. I felt that he would call me so Mom would not be within hearing range.

Afterward, while she got dressed, the doctor told me he was going change her medication again to see if it had been causing her memory problems and personality changes. I felt as if a ten-ton weight had been lifted off my shoulders. I prayed that the medication change would return Mom to her normal self again.

Joe and I watched, waited, and prayed that we would see some improvement after she had been on the new medication for a while. I believe that because we wanted so badly to see positive changes in her, we seemed to ignore the problems.

About two months after the Vegas trip, my mother had an automobile accident. It had not been her fault; she was hit from behind while turning into our street. Several times I accompanied Mom to nearby locations. During those short trips, I began to worry about her driving. Most of the time she seemed to drive normally, but there were times when her driving scared me to death. Mom would pull out in front of people or cut them off. Joe and I had tried talking to her about giving up her license, but she refused to listen. She informed us that her doctor would tell her if she should not drive and that we had no right to tell her if she could drive or not. After all, she owned her car and had a driver's license. Joe and I just kept hoping she would get better and her driving would improve.

After Mom's accident, the doctor ran a CAT scan that showed no injuries. At that time, the doctor urged that we consider taking away her car keys. This was difficult because the police did not charge her with the accident. Someone had hit her from behind as she was making a turn. We knew in our hearts that she may have stopped with no warning, or perhaps she did not signal, but we could not be sure. Regardless of the cause of Mom's problems, this accident proved to us that she had become a danger on the road to herself and others. We did not want to wait until someone was injured or killed before we dealt with the issue.

Joe and I were intelligent people, but we had no idea what we should do. Did we have the right to take her car keys away? At times Mom still seemed like her old self again, but other times we were not so sure. For years my mother never thought twice about getting in her car and taking a long trip alone or with a friend.

I would say this was one of the most difficult times for us. My mother had taught me how to drive many years ago. Now I would have to help her learn to live without driving. I could feel her pain and dismay in knowing something was going wrong with her that she had no control over. She must have been so frightened. I tried to put myself in her situation. There were times when she knew exactly what was going on, and then her mind shut down and the confusion set in. If I were in her place, I would hate to feel my independence slipping away. It was killing me to do this to her; I felt like I was torturing my own mother. What kind of horrible daughter was I? I knew it was for her own protection, but that did not stop the feelings.

The time had come for us to make some decisions, but I could not make that decision alone. Joe and I called my brother, Robert, and told him what had happened. We agreed that she had to stop driving. We were all concerned about her accident, her loss of memory, and her confusion. I told them they had to tell her, because I could not handle what felt like changing places with Mom. I found it too difficult placing restrictions upon her.

The next day I relented. Joe and I made plans to talk to Mom about her driving. It was not fair to place all that responsibility on Joe. We sat Mom down and tried to reason with her. The problem was that Mom did not think anything was wrong. First she became angry, then she forgot what we had said, and then she agreed to stop driving. Joe even went out and bought her roses to tell her how sorry we were about it. Just when we thought we settled everything, she forgot every word we had said and wanted her keys again. Then the whole process started again. She always loved Joe and never blamed him for any of this. From the look in her eyes, it was clear she blamed me, perhaps even detested me for doing this to her.

After several days of repeating the entire conversation about her not driving, we realized our methods were not working. We finally put her keys away. When she requested her keys, we asked her where she wanted to go and drove her there. The saddest part of participating in this was seeing how angry and sad she was when she was her old self. Then she seemed to fade away and not care. My heart would break after seeing that glimmer of my mother fade in and out of reality. Now she could not drive the car that she had bought for herself.

A week after we had taken Mom's car keys away from her, she came out of her bedroom with an old green spiral notebook in her hand. I could see she was her old self that day, and I was worried that she would start an argument about her driving again. Instead, she gave Joe the green book. Inside she had written down what she wanted to leave everyone when she died. She told me she wanted to talk to Joe alone, so I left the room. As I did, she was looking at Joe with such love and affection. I could see that she understood what she wanted to do at that moment but wondered if she would even remember the next day. She glanced at me to see if I had left the room yet and shot an angry, distrustful look my way. Later I found out that she told Joe that she wanted him to have her car.

The next day, Joe had her sign over the papers for the car. We thought that having it in his name would be best if she were to get worse. We promised her to use the car only to take her where she wanted to go. We kept that promise until she left our home.

I often wondered how I would feel if someone told me I could no longer drive a car. I know exactly what she must have felt during her lucid moments. She must have had so much anger and resentment toward us, and I think she mostly blamed me. I could see in the way she looked at me that she was thinking, *"I've done so much for you and your family. How could you do this to me?"* I could not blame her. I felt the same way. Later I would come to realize this was all part of the disease. At the time, I did not understand that.

In June 1992, my son Matt graduated from high school. Fortunately, Mom had a good day. We even had an enjoyable dinner out with the entire family. Matt was going to take the summer off before moving to Cedar City to attend the University. I do not know what I would have done during that summer if he had not been around. She loved spending time with Matt and his friends; no matter how bad she got, they seemed to keep her in good spirits.

Soon my last child would be leaving the nest. This gave me another reason to be sad. I had always "pulled myself up by my bootstraps" and gone on with my life no matter what. Now I felt less and less able to do that. At work, the company had begun talking about moving our department to Phoenix. This would have eliminated many jobs in the computer areas where both Joe and I worked. As a Team Leader, in middle management, my staff expected me to tell them everything. I would have, if I had known anything. Unfortunately, I had no idea what decisions were being made by upper management. As far as I knew, both Joe's and my jobs were in jeopardy, too. My stress level increased daily.

Since Tonya and Josh, my older son, had moved out of the house, Matt had been especially dedicated to both my mother and me. I have always felt that God gave me Matt to help me survive my mother's illness and to be there for her when she started forgetting things. He always spent so much time with her, and he certainly had more patience than I did.

One incident will remain in my memory forever. Matt had been alone in the kitchen with Mom. He told me she stood by the microwave pushing buttons and told him that she could not remember how to work it. He patiently helped her set the timer to warm her tea. When he finished Mom looked at him and said, "Something bad is happening to my mind." She hit herself on her head with the palm of her hand as she spoke to him. He told her that everyone forgets things sometimes, including him, but he knew she did not believe it. Matt told me later how sad it made him feel to see her so worried.

While the children were growing up, Mom often played the card game "Kings in the Corner" with them. One night, not long after his graduation, Matt asked Mom to play the game with him. As they sat playing, Matt noticed she did not deal the cards, so he did. As they began to play, he saw that she seemed to go blank. The game they had played hundreds of times before had gone from her mind. He tried to continue the game, but she just looked at him as if she did not even know who he was. It frightened him. He put the cards away and took Mom into her room. Every night before Matt would go out with his friends, he made a point to go in and give Grandma a kiss goodnight. He would sit and talk to her, even if for just a few minutes.

After taking Grandma to her room, Matt came to me and told me what had happened. I did not let him know, but I had seen this happen a few times myself. Her blank states always seemed to pass, so I told him she was just getting older and this was probably a sign of that happening. We did not know what the problem was, but somehow accepting that explanation made it easier.

When Mom had problems or forgot something, Matt would take time to explain. Now that would be my job. I was not sure I could handle that. The summer after his graduation was the beginning of Mom's plunge into Alzheimer's. We did not know it then but the disease was taking root. I worried about being alone with her, but I was glad that the children did not have to go through this disease with my mother. It was difficult enough when they would visit and wonder if she knew who they were. Tonya said it was just like her great-grandmother. She had been about seven when her great-grandmother became ill and could not remember her. It had made a terrible impression upon her young mind. Now, again, someone so close to her all these years did not know who she was.

In October of 1993, while Joe was away on a business trip, things began to get worse. A lack of sleep had left me exhausted. I had been driving all over town to do both Mom's errands and my own. Now I was doing all the cooking and cleaning and still working full-time with considerable stress at my job. Mom seemed more agitated than usual, and she was not sleeping well. Her medicine caused nightmares. She would either scream or walk around the house in a panic. More than once I found her standing over me while I slept, and I was now becoming afraid of her. I started locking my door. I knew if she were the Mom I grew up with, I had nothing to fear, but this new person disturbed me. I did not know what she was capable of doing in a half-sleep state.

*   *   *

I expected to find Joe and Mom both upset from the incident that occurred earlier at Neighborhood House. Instead, I found both of them sitting calmly watching television. Joe had cooked dinner and had something warming for me in the kitchen.

As we got dressed for bed, I asked Joe what happened when he went to pick up Mom.

"When I arrived, they had things pretty well under control. One of the staff was sitting with her doing a craft."

"Did they say anything about what happened?"

"They said she was very upset and convinced that someone was going to put her in jail. Even after the bus drove off she seemed to think her friends were being kidnapped. They had to divert her mind to crafts in order to get her calmed down."

"On the way home, she didn't seem to have any problems?" I asked.

"No, she seemed a bit jittery but other than that she was okay." Joe replied.

"I'm very concerned that they will not let her stay at Neighborhood House much longer. A few more incidents like this one and they may tell us that they are not equipped to handle her," I said.

"We will deal with that when the time comes. With the way things are going, we need to take one day at a time. That is all we can do," Joe said.

CHAPTER 8

February 1993 had been a very difficult month at work. I tried to concentrate on my job but my mind kept going to my mother. Her problems at Neighborhood House had been on the increase. I wondered how long it would be before they would tell me she could no longer stay there during the day. What would we do then?

I was going through my purse and came across one of the credit card bills for Tonya's wedding and realized how glad I was that she had not been home to watch her beloved grandmother deteriorate mentally. They had such a close relationship and did so many things together. I hated to shop but Tonya and Mom loved it. They traveled together and talked together for hours at a time. I was so glad that she had the chance to share that special day with her grandma.

*   *   *

In May of 1992 I helped Tonya plan her August wedding that was a mixture of heaven and hell for me. Most of the time, I took Mom shopping with us. I enjoyed looking around at wedding dresses, but Mom would get agitated easily and want to go home before we were done. Because Tonya had not been around her much, she did not understand the way Mom was acting and I could not tell her at such a happy time in her life.

Tonya enjoyed trying on dress after dress. After the first few shopping trips, I dreaded taking Mom along because she would get confused and would ask to go home. So I tried to plan the shopping trips when Matt or Joe would be home to stay with Mom.

Mom had a good friend she met while working at the church. Lisa would occasionally come to visit and take her out for the day. She and Mom had been working on a wedding gift for Tonya for months. One day Lisa called to ask Mom to go to lunch but I picked up the phone. Before I called Mom to the phone, Lisa said that she could see a real change in Mom over the past few months.

"We are sewing a quilt for Tonya's wedding gift. When we started the quilt in December, your mom was so excited about it, but by spring she began having problems concentrating on what she was doing. I thought it may have been the medication she was taking, but the last two times your mother and I came to my house to work on the quilt, it was clear that she could barely concentrate on it or even understand what to do next," she said.

"I know, she is having problems," I said.

"Have you had her checked?"

"Yes, the doctor has examined her many times. He has changed her medication hoping that would help. They even did a CAT scan after her accident. Everything looked fine."

"Have you ever considered she may have Alzheimer's disease? My aunt had it for years and your mother's symptoms are very similar." Lisa sounded sad.

"What makes you think that?"

"I think it would be better if your doctor explained it to you. It's far too complicated and I don't know all the particulars about it."

"Thanks, I'll call and ask him about it."

Just then Mom walked into the room and I handed the phone over to her.

Lisa was about ten years younger than Mom, but they enjoyed many of the same things. I knew Lisa was concerned about what was happening to Mom and wanted to help. I have to admit I really did not think much about the possibility of Mom's having Alzheimer's disease mostly because I did not know much about it at that time. After all, I felt sure that the doctors would have told me if they suspected something like that. Certainly the CAT scan would have shown something wrong with her brain. Mom had just been to see her doctor two weeks before to follow up on her medication, and the doctor had said nothing to me at that time. However, because of Lisa's phone call, I decided to call him when the wedding was over.

Mom and I went shopping to find something special for her to wear to the wedding. She seemed to enjoy being the center of attention as I helped her try on dress after dress. Once we found her a beautiful dress for the wedding we set up appointments to have our hair and nails done. She also seemed to enjoy being pampered, but I was not sure she always knew why we were doing it.

Tonya continued with her wedding arrangements at the ski lodge where she worked and where the wedding would be held. I went along with her once to help order the food for the wedding. After our shopping trips for her wedding dress, Tonya knew something was not right with her grandma and tried to do as much as possible on her own. I felt very sad about that. She was my only daughter and I wanted to be more involved, but I felt guilty leaving Mom at home with Joe while I helped Tonya get through the shopping stages of her wedding.

Then the big day arrived. Mom looked beautiful in her new dress. Joe and the boys were so handsome in their tuxes. I even felt like I looked nice, despite being overweight. We had reserved a block of rooms at the ski lodge where the wedding and reception were to be held. My brother, Robert, had come from Wisconsin and Joe's parents had come from Florida for the wedding. Joe's sister, Angela, and her three children were there, too.

Tonya and her two maids of honor, Lori and Jill, were in the room that would later be the honeymoon suite. Lori and Jill had stayed the night before and were helping Tonya prepare for the wedding. When we arrived, Jill answered the door. I heard Tonya's voice and glanced up to the loft where she stood. She looked like an elegant picture in her bridal gown. Her father and I were so proud. Mom did not say much, but she did smile. As the photographer took pictures, I could see that Mom was confused by all the activity going on around her.

The day was perfect, sunny and cloudless with a slight breeze. Mountains covered with huge pine trees made the backdrop for the ceremony. When the music played, the notes seemed to transcend the ski lodge deck and move through the trees. Tonya and Mike were a vision. She looked like a princess and Mike, her prince. We called them our Barbie and Ken wedding set because they resembled the dolls.

After the reception, Joe and I went to our own room. My brother had a large suite with two bedrooms; he offered to have Mom stay with him. It was delightful not to worry about Mom for one night. I had tried to forget everything that was happening at home and focus on the wedding, and on Joe.

The next day at breakfast, Robert told me that Mom had gotten up at 5:00 a.m. and wanted to go to church. It was Sunday, so she was right about church. He did not understand why she was up that early and determined to go to church. He knew she had been having some problems, but now he was seeing a glimpse of them first-hand. We enjoyed having breakfast with our friends and family before making the trip home. Elizabeth and Salvador came home with us for a week.

While Elizabeth was at our home, she spent a lot of time with Mom. Even when Mom would look blank, Elizabeth patiently sat and talked to her. After a week, they left for Florida, and things returned to the way they had been. I no longer had others taking time with Mom. Once again, Joe and I had to take over Mom's care.

It seemed to me that with every passing month, Mom lost a little more of herself. Now that the wedding was over, I called the doctor and learned that he was on vacation. Since Mom had become so uncomfortable going to the doctor, I did not want to take her to someone new. When her doctor returned, he changed her medication by phone and said to call back to make an appointment for the first part of December, which I did. He said that he would evaluate the effects of the medication and assess her condition at that time.

We continued to cope as best we could. Sometimes the new medication made her lethargic. I hated that. It bothered me that the drugs made her sleep more than usual and increased her confusion. I just did not understand what the doctor was doing, but I trusted him. Because my brother and his wife were both Biomedical Engineers, I called and talked to Robert several times. He told me to look up her medications in the drug interaction book I had bought. I told him what the book said and asked for his opinion. I wanted to sound informed when I questioned the doctor about my findings.

Once Mom's doctor examined her again, I told him what I had found in the book and how it applied to Mom's actions. He agreed to take her off one of the medicines and once again told me to keep him updated on Mom's reaction. I agreed.

Matt started college in September of 1992. Matt, Mom, and I drove him and his belongings to Cedar City. Mom dozed off several times and we chatted about incidental things. I would let her start the conversation and then respond to her comments. It was easier that way. If I started to talk, she could not always understand what I said.

When we arrived at our hotel in Cedar City, I decided not to leave Mom in the car. I was worried that she might leave the car and walk away. I got out of the car and walked over to open Mom's door.

"Why are we here?" she asked.

"This is where Josh goes to college, remember? Now Matt will be going to school here, too," I said. She did not seem to understand what I was saying.

When we arrived, we called Josh who gave us directions to the house into which Matt would be moving. Several young men helped us take the furniture and boxes out of the van. While Mom sat in the living room, I helped with the unpacking.

Whenever Josh and Matt stopped to talk to her, Mom seemed confused about the whole thing. She did not seem to mind when they hugged her, but she did not seem to recognize Josh. The change of surroundings seemed to make her uncomfortable. When Josh asked me what was wrong, I said that Matt would explain when they were alone. Mom had practically raised Josh for the first few months of his life when my back was injured. Now she barely recognized him. I knew he was devastated.

After we returned to the hotel and unpacked, Mom and I drove to a fast-food place and had a hamburger. We returned to the hotel for a rest and later decided to go for a relaxing walk. Mom loved to take walks, and I liked them because they always seemed to calm her down. The most beautiful red-rock mountains surround Cedar City. Walking would help us unwind after our long ride. While we walked, I tried to get Mom to remember things. I mentioned how she used to rock Josh in the rocking chair and sing to him. She and Dad loved being around the boys when they were little. I talked about how Josh and Matt used to roll around and play as toddlers. I talked about their first few Christmases when their grandpa would come in with his big red bag filled with gifts. Occasionally I would see a spark of remembrance in her eyes, but it saddened me to see the confusion that followed.

Over the past few months, her days had changed from about 80 percent recognition to 40 percent. I had watched as she went from an extremely intelligent, well read, organized woman to a woman who could not read and could only scribble words that made little sense. I wondered how much worse things could get.

That evening, I helped Mom get dressed for dinner. I told the boys I would treat them to dinner at the Holiday Inn before we left the next day. When the boys arrived, we sat and chatted a bit until I finished putting on my make-up. They made a fuss over Mom, which lifted her spirits. Then Josh let Mom put her arm through his as we walked to the restaurant together. No matter what she remembered at the time, she always loved attention.

Matt had whispered to me on the way to the restaurant that he could see how much Mom had gone downhill since Tonya's wedding only a month before. I did not think she had changed that much. Both boys had been in the wedding party, but they had been so busy that they did not really have much time alone with their grandma. Now, however, they were alone with her and attempting to make conversation. At times she would get frustrated because she could not remember a word, and they would say something to get her mind off it.

We all pitched in to help Mom at the salad bar and again when we ordered dinner. We had to be non-intrusive about the way we helped her because she usually wanted to do things on her own. Mom seemed to have a good time. Josh took me aside and told me how sorry he was that Grandma was forgetting so much. I told him not to worry. Because Mom was close by, I did not want to get into a lengthy conversation about it. After all, there was nothing they could do about it.

We told the boys we would meet them for breakfast before we left the next morning. Mom and I gave them big kisses and hugs and went back to our room. I helped Mom change her clothes and take her medication, and then I settled her into a chair to watch television while I changed. Once I finished brushing my teeth, I returned to the room to find Mom standing at the window looking out into the dark.

"That was a pleasant dinner, wasn't it, Mom?" I asked.

"Who were those people?"

"They were your grandsons, Mom. Don't you remember?" I had familiar tears in my eyes.

"Okay," she said.

I knew she had forgotten the two boys who had been the center of her life for fifteen years. After she went to bed, I laid awake for hours, worried that she might wake up during the night. Finally I realized that she probably could not figure out the security latch and let myself drift off to sleep.

Our trip home was so depressing. Now all three of my children were out on their own. I felt very alone that day. I left a large piece of my heart behind with Matt and Josh that weekend. I was happy for them but sad to be so far away from them. I also knew that Mom did not really understand that Matt would be in college. It would be yet another question I did not know how to answer for her.

All that went through my mind on the way home was: Why would God take so many memories from Mom? Why was God taking my mother away from me, too? She had always done everything she could for everyone else. I knew that thinking about myself was selfish, but I was angry. My children were gone, and now God wanted to take my mother's mind. The only lifeline I had left was Joe. If not for him, I would have been tempted to drive off a mountain top that day.

*   *   *

I jumped when the phone on my desk rang. My thoughts had taken me to another time and place. That seemed to be happening more often. Perhaps it was an escape or wanting to remember the days when my mother was an intelligent, vibrant woman. My mother had now become my child. At times, this feeling overwhelmed me. I had always gone to her with my problems, and we had talked, sometimes for hours, about the children. Now all that wisdom she used to impart was gone. I was losing everyone, or at least that is the way I felt.

CHAPTER 9

Tonya was about to have my first grandchild. As her due date grew closer, I decided to look through a chest of my children's baby clothes that I had saved. I came across some booties, blankets and caps that my mother and grandmother had knitted for them. It was more than I could take. I was thrilled to be a grandmother for the first time, but wondered if my mother would even understand that she was to become a great-grandmother. Would she even recognize Tonya and Mike? So many questions filled me with sadness. I remembered the last big family gathering.

*　　*　　*

In November of 1992, the family came to our house to celebrate Thanksgiving dinner. Mom had always been the main cook for our holiday meals but had reached a point where she just could not cook anymore. She could not remember how to put foods together or how to measure amounts for recipes. These days she became confused at the most simple tasks.

Since I had taken over the cooking duties, meals had become more simple and quick. The wonderful recipes made from scratch and never really measured were now gone. I had attempted using her recipes, but the pies did not taste the same at all. Since my schedule at work required that I be there such long hours, I did not have the time to spend baking. I was lucky to get the turkey in the oven and dinner on the table.

Because I could tell that Mom wanted to help by the way she wandered around the kitchen, I decided to ask her to make the gravy. I figured that since I would be right there, I could help her if she looked like she could not handle the task. She looked at me, looked around, and finally went to the freezer and took out the ice cubes. I did not make a big deal about it. I just said, "That's a good idea, you can fill the glasses with ice for the iced tea." That seemed fine with her. Tonya helped her get started and work her way around the table. Seeing Mom looking so confused upset Tonya and me, but we continued so as not to spoil the day. My cooking did not have the special touch of prior Thanksgivings. There were no homemade pies, candied yams, or even flour on her nose, but we were together. Times were changing slowly, but little did I know just how much.

The day went well but I could see the concern in Tonya's face. Mom did not seem to know us half the time. Tonya took me aside and asked me how long she had been like this. I told her it had been getting worse since her wedding. She said it reminded her of Mary, Mom's mother.

"I wonder if she will forget me like Grandma Mary did?" Tonya held back tears. That memory had always been difficult for her.

"I don't know, honey. Only God knows that. We just have to take it one day at a time." I patted her on the shoulder but felt like crying myself.

After Thanksgiving, Joe and I wanted to start shopping for Christmas gifts. Except for work, we had not been out of the house much since the wedding. We decided to spend that entire Saturday shopping. We thought Mom should also get out of the house for awhile and decided to take her with us. I could help her do some Christmas shopping and then we could all go to lunch afterward. Mom seemed fine as I helped her get ready. After I made sure we had everything we needed, we took off.

The stores were already crowded. I had a list for Mom and one for Joe and me. I knew that would help us get done faster. When it came to helping Mom with her shopping, I had to guess what she wanted and for whom. I made sure she bought a gift for her friend Lisa and the nuns at the church where she had worked. Then I helped her get something for each child. I did not get anything big, just something she could afford to give them. They all knew the situation and would understand.

As we walked around from store to store, either Joe or I had to watch Mom carefully. She would wander and become disoriented at times. I had to help her make out her checks for her gifts and hoped she could remember how to sign them. At times she did not even know what a check was. In those cases, I just made out my own check and paid for it myself. When I had to stand in line for my gifts, Joe took care of Mom and made sure she was okay. We had to make sure she did not get lost in the crowds.

When we finished shopping, we put the packages in the car and went to The Olive Garden Restaurant to have lunch. Mom had always enjoyed their soup and salad. We had done well. We had bought nearly everything on our lists, and Mom just followed along not really causing any problems. When we sat and started to look through the menu, I noticed Mom had her hand over the menu, not looking at it at all.

"Do you know what you want Mom?" I asked.

"I want a one of—" She could not think of the words.

"Would you like soup and a salad, then maybe a dessert?" I asked.

"Okay," she said quietly.

"Well, we got a lot accomplished, didn't we? Did you enjoy yourself today Mom?"

"No, you spent all my money," she said.

I gasped in shock. "What do you mean Mom? I only helped you buy presents for your friends and spent my own money for my gifts."

I was so hurt. My heart was pounding like a sledge hammer on metal. Joe held my hand and said, "Marie, she didn't mean it. You know she didn't mean it." I did not listen to him. She did mean it. I knew she did.

"So you didn't enjoy shopping today at all?" I could not seem to stop myself from asking.

"No. I didn't like all those—" and again she could not think of the words. I wondered how she could always find the words that hurt me. They seemed to come to her without any problem at all.

We ate our lunch, but I could not forget how she had hurt me. I ate my food so fast that I nearly became ill.

When we returned home, I just took the gifts out of the bags and threw them across the room one at a time. Then I ran into my room and slammed the door like a spoiled child. I cried so hard I could not hold my lunch down.

Poor Joe, first he had to calm down my mother and try to explain it all to her. He told me she just had that blank expression on her face like she had no idea why I did that. I know now that she did not understand why I lost my temper, and for that matter, neither did I.

After he cleaned up the gifts and got Mom settled, he came into our room. He looked at me with a half disgusted, half sympathetic look on his face. He held my shoulders in his hands and looked me straight in the eye and said. "Marie, you know that wasn't your mother saying those words. Why did you get angry?"

I felt even worse than I had before. Now I was losing his respect, too. I looked down at the floor, unable to face him, and said. "She hates me. She has always hated me. I'm a terrible daughter. No matter what I ever do, it won't be good enough for her."

My mother's words were like a knife that left a bleeding wound in my heart. She did not trust me. Joe just held me in his arms and let me cry again. This began to happen several times a week. I was constantly being hurt by comments she made. Instead of dealing with it like an adult, I felt like a child who was being punished by her mother's words. I would go to my room and shut the door and feel guilty that I was not doing a good job of caring for her. Thoughts went through my mind about why my mother hated me. I wondered what the doctors would find when they examined her.

I had been taking notes of her behavior to give the doctor information about her condition. During that week, Mom's brother Steven called and asked if he could take her on a trip back to visit relatives in Pennsylvania. I could barely handle everything that was happening at home now. I tried to explain about her condition and that I did not think she should be traveling now. From his experience with his mother-in-law who had had dementia, he felt he could handle anything that may come up.

I told him I was taking her to the doctor for a check-up that week. At that time I would ask her doctor if he thought that traveling would be okay for her. Then I told Steven when I found out I would call him back and let him know. I was a wreck about it. As much as I could have used a break from her, I would worry about her every day. It did not matter if she were with Steven or not. He may not realize how she would wander off or say strange things. I would leave it up to the doctor. After all he knew a lot more than I did, right? It was my way of coping with the situation. I had always felt if I ignored a problem, it would go away. It was not the way I should have handled it. It was the same self-protection mechanism I had used from the time I was very young.

In December 1992, Mom's trip to the doctor had been uneventful. I had taken in some information for the doctor to read before her exam. It explained, in detail, the problems Mom had been experiencing. The list included loss of memory that affected her writing checks, balancing her checkbook, and cooking. I wrote about her difficulty dressing herself, how she put her clothes on backward or inside out, and would wear summer clothes in the cold of winter. I also explained about how I had to tell her to shower. I noted the problems she had finding words to complete a sentence or a thought. She had problems with days, time, and knowing where she was. These days, I had to go with her any time she left the house. I also noted the problems she had putting things somewhere and forgetting where they were. Her moods had been changing. She would be calm then get very angry for no reason. She did not seem to want to do anything she had once done, like reading, gardening or crafts.

During the appointment, I asked the doctor about the trip Steven wanted to take her on. He asked me if Steven had any experience with the problems Mom was having. I told him how Steven had cared for his mother-in-law when she was suffering from dementia. The doctor said as long as he kept a close eye on her to make certain she did not wander off, it was probably okay for her to go. I had hoped he would say she should not go and did ask him if he was sure she would be all right. I did not like to discuss Mom's problems in front of her so I called the doctor after the appointment to follow up. He told me when she returned he wanted to set her up with a psychiatrist he knew who handled dementia-type diseases. He thought she should be checked out. I could not get any more information out of him. He said he needed to get the results back from the psychiatrist before he could diagnose the problem. I had been sure he would have some answers after this visit, but I still had no idea what was going through his mind. I thought she was becoming senile like her mother.

After the doctor's appointment, I called Steven to talk about the trip. I was afraid for both Steven and Mom and knew he was not aware of her recent changes. I decided to try to talk the situation over with him and see how he felt. Steven said he could handle the situation and seemed determined that everything would be fine, but I was not so sure. Steven loved his sister dearly and would take wonderful care of her no matter what. He was a far more patient person than I was. Maybe it would be a good thing for both of us to have a rest from each other.

I became concerned as we packed her clothes for the trip. I packed her medicine and wrote notes about time and the dose of each pill she needed to take. I could not let her do it herself anymore. Steven would have to take on this responsibility for her.

Most of the time Mom seemed to know she was going somewhere with Steven, her brother. Other times, she wanted to know why she was going somewhere and where she was going. It made me feel guilty letting her go. It was like I did not want her around. I guess a part of me was glad she was going, but another part of me felt like a mother whose child was going on their first sleep over. It worried me that she might be afraid or not know what was happening to her.

Life stayed busy for me. Decorating the house, writing Christmas cards, and making plans for Christmas dinner left me little free time to think. Despite being busy, I worried about Mom's pending trip. Time pasted too quickly; the trip was only two days away now. I had to get all her things washed and packed for her. She was excited about taking a trip with Steven. She loved him so much.

Steven has always been a fun person to have around. I knew he would be good for Mom right now. I knew I was not and had been having a hard time cracking my usual smile lately. I did not want those around me to know how I really felt. I maintained that facade, the happy-go-lucky one that everyone expected. Inside was a whole different thing. My heart was breaking as I watched my mother's mind deteriorate, but I knew I had to keep going for her sake. She really needed me now. I had to be there for her.

Steven arrived in Utah, stayed a few days, and then they left with Mom. In my heart, I knew she would be fine with Steven. He would take wonderful care of her but she had been going through some very strange moods lately. She could change suddenly and become angry or frightened. I worried but could do nothing at this point. I went about celebrating Christmas with the rest of my family.

The children came for Christmas Day and we enjoyed the time together. I knew Mom and Steven were going to visit Robert and his family first. After that, they would continue on to St. Louis, then drive to Pennsylvania and Maryland to visit other family members. I tried to keep my mind on my children and their Christmas, but it was difficult. My mind would often deviate to Mom. I had marked all her medications, and written down everything she needed, but was that enough? Did I forget anything important?

Two days after Christmas, in the evening, I received a call from my cousin in Maryland. My mother was very upset about her purse and her money. She was accusing Steven of taking her money, just as she had done with me during our Christmas shopping trip. They could not calm her down and thought it might help if I talked to her. When they put her on the phone, I could barely understand what she was saying to me. I did not let my voice show how worried I was. Instead I calmly said, "Hi Mom. Are you having a good time?" She tried to mumble something about her money.

"This is Mom (she had been calling me Mom for some time now). You are at Fran's house? Are you having a nice time?" I repeated questions to her in a calm voice. Before long she became more concerned with answering my questions and forgot to be angry with Steven or that she had even been upset. I talked to her for quite a while, until she totally calmed down. Eventually my cousin got back on the phone and thanked me. She said if I ever needed to talk, I could call her. Of course, I did not want to bother anyone with my problems. I could deal with things myself, or so I thought.

A week went by and Mom was due to fly back to Utah from St. Louis by herself. I noticed my hands shaking as I drove to the airport to pick up Mom. I arrived very early to wait for the plane to arrive. When the passengers began to disembark, I waited patiently for Mom to come through the gate. The plane was nearly empty by the time I finally saw Mom. I knew immediately something was not right. Two flight attendants came out with Mom. Each attendant had one of her arms walking down the runway with her. I ran over to her and started to hug Mom.

"Are you all right? Is she all right? What happened?" I asked.

One attendant took me aside and said that my mother had gotten very agitated, difficult to handle. They had changed her seat with a man near where the attendants worked so they could manage the situation.

"She is still confused. I think she will be better now that someone she knows is with her."

The attendants left and I hugged Mom for a long time. She seemed to calm down. I sat her down in a chair for a few minutes, held her hand, and talked quietly to her about her trip and Steven. It seemed to make her feel better. When she calmed down enough, we went to get her bag and go home. I will never forget how frightened she looked as she debarked that plane. I felt very guilty for allowing her to be on that plane alone.

Once Mom returned home and began to settle in, things seemed to calm down. She remembered where she was and became comfortable again but she was having more problems. I started to worry about leaving her at home alone when we were working. Since Matt had gone to college, no one would be with her. I had asked her friend Lisa and our neighbors, Susan and Ned, to come and check on her once in awhile, but I still worried constantly that she would wander away or hurt herself.

The first week of January 1993, Joe and I left for work in the morning as we did each day but we never expected the snow would accumulate over a foot. The roads became unpassable. I kept calling our house but there was no answer. I was a total basket case after my third try. Where was Mom? Why didn't she answer the phone? Had she gone outside in that weather? Was she freezing to death as I tried to get her on the phone? Finally I was able to reach my neighbor who had been out shoveling her driveway. I asked her if she could check on Mom. She went right over to the house when we hung up. About fifteen minutes later, she called me back.

"I knocked on the door and did not get an answer but I could see her looking out the window at me. I don't know whether she didn't recognize me or what, but I called out to her several times. She just stood there and peaked at me through the curtains. Maybe our heavy coats made it difficult to recognize me. Do you want me to do anything else?" Susan asked.

"Did she seem like she was sick or hurt?" I asked.

"No, not at all. She just would not answer the door," Susan said.

"No, I think the plows are cleaning the streets here now. I can probably get home within a couple of hours. Could you just kind of watch the house so she does not go out without a coat and freeze to death?"

"Sure, I will go and check on her every fifteen minutes or have one of the kids make sure she is still in there."

I thanked Susan and hoped everything would be all right until Joe and I could dig out and get home. It took about three hours more to get home. My stress level was through the roof. Between the terrible road conditions and the worry about Mom, I could feel myself developing a migraine headache.

When we finally arrived, I opened the garage door. I could see my Mom had the door from the house to the garage opened and was sitting in the rocking chair looking out at us. More worried than angry, I bounded into the house and asked if she was all right. I will never forget the look on her face. It was so peaceful. She said, very clearly, "Those beautiful ladies in long white dresses kept singing and going into that place up there." She pointed to the attic crawl space, still covered with the wooden door.

I was confused. "Why didn't you answer the phone Mom?" I asked.

"They were trying to steal my papers." She said.

"Who Mom?" I asked.

"Someone out there." She pointed to the door. I knew she meant Susan. She had not recognized her.

"But Mom, why didn't you answer the phone?" I asked again.

"They were bad people trying to get my papers." She said again.

I decided I would not keep asking because she did not understand what I meant anyway. From that day on, I knew I had to do something. Joe and I could not leave her alone anymore. The next day, I called the doctor and told him what had happened. That was when he had me schedule the appointment with the psychiatrist.

To this day I wonder if Mom really did see angels. Had they been taking care of her while she was alone? I had to believe that she had a glimpse of a beautiful place better than earth. I hoped those ladies in long white dresses in that other dimension kept her safe and happy as they sang to her. I have to believe that so I do not go crazy thinking about it.

It was right after that incident that Joe and I found and enrolled her in Neighborhood House. I knew I had to make sure Mom would be safe during the day when Joe and I were at work. We were very lucky that she had not hurt herself.

*   *   *

Mom had come into the room looking for me. She looked at the tiny cap and sweater, and to my amazement said, "My mother made that." I was so shocked that she seemed to know this fact. With all the things she had forgotten lately, there was still an occasional recognition or memory that would find its way to the surface. With her recognizing that her mother had knitted these baby clothes, I felt a small glimmer of hope. I wished that I could turn back time so she could remember everything again, and that I would have another chance to be a better daughter.

Part II

Decisions

CHAPTER 10

All during the month of February 1993, Joe had problems driving Mom to Neighborhood House. One evening, out of concern for Mom, he told me about his recent experiences.

"Any morning I take a different route or the traffic is especially heavy, she gets very anxious. I try to explain but it rarely does any good. I worry that she may try to jump out of the car someday," Joe said.

"Mom has a very difficult time opening the door on the van. As you know, we have to help her on and off with her seat belt and opening the door. I think it is very unlikely she could do that." I put my hand on his shoulder to reassure him.

"I have to wait until I drive up to Neighborhood House and then tell her again where we are. She seems to improve once we walk inside even though she rarely remembers the others' names," Joe said.

"I have the same problem any time I drive her around on errands. We just have to try to keep her calm. I find changing the subject helps. Talk about the music on the radio or something in the van. That seems to take her mind off where she is going. It doesn't always work but it has helped on occasion."

Even though Neighborhood House helped us in some ways, there were other problems that developed. Most of the time she would do very well there, but on several occasions she became paranoid about the strangest things. We had known, from everything the manager had told us, that this would not be a permanent solution. I tried not to think about what may be coming next. I only planned a week at a time these days. Our anniversary would be in a few days, and I wanted to plan something special for that day if at all possible.

On February 14, 1993, I completed plans for an enjoyable anniversary dinner at home. Unlike our first years of marriage, we no longer had mini-vacations or went to fancy restaurants. We had promised ourselves when we married to make our anniversary romantic and special every year. Things change and so did this promise. It had become important to make Mom feel safe and secure than to keep our promise to each other. Joe and I just accepted the changes. We felt more comfortable at home than if we had tried to leave my mother with someone else or attempted to take her out to eat. These days Mom would get confused when we took her out to eat anyway.

I prepared a roast and set the table to look special. It would not be romantic, but at least it would be an enjoyable evening. I wanted one uneventful dinner, but I became more tense as the evening drew near. Mom clung to me all day as if something were bothering her. Finally I decided to take a break. I checked the roast and went into the living room to watch television. I knew Mom would follow me and I thought she might just sit with me for a while.

I jumped as the buzzer went off in the kitchen. As much as I wanted to just sit and relax, I needed to finish our anniversary dinner. As I looked over at Mom, who had dozed off again, she looked so sweet, small, and helpless. I got up quietly and went into the kitchen to make mashed potatoes. Mom had taught me all I knew about cooking. I could not come close to cooking the way she once did, but when I had time and energy, I could cook a decent meal. As I lit the match for the candles, I thought about our anniversary and knew just how blessed I was to have found Joe.

When Joe came home, he could see the dozen red roses he had sent and a beautifully set table. "Something smells great." He held me in his arms and gave me a big anniversary kiss. "How was your Mom today?" he asked.

"Actually it was a pretty quiet day. I took Mom for a walk earlier and I think it wore her out. She fell asleep. So overall, a mellow day," I said.

He went in and changed, then woke Mom up, and we had a very pleasant dinner. For one night, things were calm. With the changes Alzheimer's disease brought about, we had learned not be expect that very often.

Most of my days had become so stressful. I just existed going from chore to chore, day after day. I barely slept and worried all the time. My life seemed like one big chore. I dreaded what tomorrow would bring so I dared not look into the future. No longer did I look forward to work or even my family. I just hoped I could make it through another day. I thought it was up to me to take care of everything. I felt responsible for taking care of Mom, my job, Joe, and the house. Instead of being grateful that Joe often helped me, I felt more guilty.

I had never been a particularly patient person, but after Mom was diagnosed with Alzheimer's disease, I began to change. No matter how much stress I felt, I only lost my temper few times, and it was more with myself than with her. I never felt that I lived up to my mother's expectations. She hated that I was overweight, and that I did not dress in fancy clothes or go to fancy restaurants for lunch. I had always been more of a casual dresser and loved fast-food places. It was difficult to ignore, I would hear some of the hurtful things that she would say but, I knew she had no idea why her words upset me. When I would see her reaction, I knew being upset was the wrong way to respond. Guilt came over me immediately if I felt the least bit angry because she did not understand why I felt that way.

I often wonder if her having this disease was God's way of testing my reaction. God knew I had no patience and was trying to teach me how to do it right. It worked. I began to take time, to give her hugs and kisses and encouragement. In my entire life, I had always been the one who wanted these things from her and never gotten them. Now the tables were turned. I was not going to treat her that way. I knew how it felt. She loved me, but sometimes I knew she did not like me much. Now I just loved her unconditionally, like a person loves a helpless child. I wanted to do the best I could for her but was not sure I knew how.

When she would sit in a chair and gaze into blankness, I could not help but wonder where her mind went. Even though I was angry with God, I had to make myself believe in a higher power. Was she seeing something that I could not see? The way I dealt with that part of her illness was to imagine her mind going into a much better place. I began to think of that place as one of unbelievable beauty. I thought of it as a form of meditation. She went beyond earth into a garden of magnificent colors and lights where she only felt happiness. Her struggles no longer existed. She had no more pain, and she floated on a soft, cloud. At least I prayed that was what she encountered in her silence.

In the afternoon of February 28, 1993, we received the call we had been waiting for. Tonya had been in labor for several hours. Her contractions were regular and close enough together, and the doctor told her to get to the hospital. Tonya said they would call us from there. We waited patiently for two hours until she called us back. She was in labor but still had a long time to go. The hospital would not admit her yet, so she asked if she could come to our house and wait since our house was a little closer to the hospital than theirs.

When Tonya and Mike arrived, I could tell she was miserable. She kept doing her breathing exercises but said she dreaded the long drive back to the hospital. She and Mike did not have very good insurance, and the hospital was not willing to admit her seemingly until the last minute before the baby's birth. Joe and I were upset but had no recourse. We decided to pack us all up and go get rooms at the Embassy Suite Hotel, right around the corner from the hospital. That way, Tonya could go back and forth until the hospital accepted her. I tried to comfort her and Mike helped her with her breathing. I packed a few things for us and we called a hotel to reserve two connecting rooms.

In one room Joe, Mom and I watched television. I had told Tonya I was there if she needed me, but I did not want to interfere with this special time between her and Mike. I think Mom knew something was not normal, and the situation agitated her. She kept saying, "I want to go to my place." I tried to tell her that her granddaughter, Tonya, was having a baby very soon. Mom wanted no part of it. She ranted and raved like a spoiled, mean child. When I took out my small address book to call someone, and she pulled it out of my hand, ripping it in half.

When Joe went in to give Mike some snacks that we had room service deliver, Mom heard Tonya's breathing and moaning.

"Who is that and what is wrong with her?" Mom asked as she pointed to Tonya. I do not think Tonya heard her, but I felt a strong need to protect her from Mom's words. Tonya would have been so sad to hear her say that. I knew she would have flashbacks to when her great-grandmother did not recognize her. I did not want to make the situation worse, so I went into the bedroom to call my other children to let them know Tonya had gone into labor while Joe tried to calm Mom down but even he had a very hard time.

Later that evening, I had to give Mom her medication. She refused to take it and even tried to throw it away. Joe asked me if he should just take Mom home. Since Joe had adopted my children and had never been there for the birth of a baby, I knew he did not want to leave. He should be able to be there for his daughter now. Knowing that Tonya wanted me there too, I decided we would tough it out together.

I could not sleep at all. Mom finally took her medication and relaxed a little. As she dozed off, I just sat on a chair and waiting for word from Tonya. Late into the night, Tonya and Mike decided it was time to go back to the hospital, this time she was admitted. Mom was more calm now but still confused. Joe and I alternated walking up and down the halls with her. She finally fell asleep on the sofa in the waiting room. I could not believe she had gone on for so long. How could someone her age have so much energy? Joe and I were both exhausted.

Early in the morning of March 1, after thirty-six hours of labor, beautiful, eight-pound, nine-ounce, Lori was born. Both mother and baby were doing fine. Dad looked excited, tired, happy, and proud. We visited Tonya and the baby, and even Mom enjoyed seeing the baby.

Once Tonya dozed off, we all went home to get some sleep. I settled Mom into her bed and Joe and I fell right asleep. For some reason, I woke up and decided to check on Mom. When I went toward her room I gasped when I saw that her door was open and her bed was empty. This was not the first time she had wandered away and I feared the consequences. I ran around the house and found no sign of her. I saw the door to the outside was open, but when I looked outside, I saw nothing. By this time, my heart was beating nearly out of my chest as I ran to get Joe.

Joe and I decided to take different directions to go look for her. I asked my neighbor to help, so we could cover many directions. After about a half hour of searching, I came back to the house to see if anyone else had any luck.

Joe and Mom were standing in the driveway with the neighbors. Joe took me aside and said, "She took off again. I found her southwest about two miles away. She said she wanted to go to her place. We thought she meant the Neighborhood House." Joe was extremely upset. "She would not get in the car with me. She didn't know who I was." He was shaking. "I finally got her to come with me but she really fought me."

"I'm so sorry honey." I patted his arm. I thanked my neighbors and went back inside. Mom was not dressed warmly, and I was afraid she may get sick, so I fixed her some hot tea. She did not want anything except to go to "Her place." Joe suggested he take her over there, and I agreed. It was only 10:30 a.m. so she could remain at Neighborhood House for the rest of the day. We were both too shaken to go back to sleep anyway. When he returned home from dropping Mom off at

Neighborhood House, he could see I had been crying since he left. "Marie, you can't keep this up. I'm losing you, too. You can't let this happen. I've always been willing to do whatever needed to be done for you and your family, but this is more than I can take. You can't hold up to this much longer. I'm calling your brother right now."

"I'll be okay. I'm just so tired and so sad." I tried to argue but had no fight left in me.

"Look at you. You just had your first grandchild and you can't stop crying. Something is wrong with this picture. You get no sleep, you work a full-time job, you just had your last child leave home, and you're not doing well. You constantly have headaches, you cry all the time. You can't do it anymore. You are destroyed over what has happened to your mother. You put up a great front to the outside world, but I know what is happening. You can't fool me."

I could do nothing but look at him. I knew that his words were true.

"I made a decision driving to Neighborhood House with your mother. We need to look at putting her somewhere with trained people to care for her. She is becoming a danger to herself. We don't know how to handle her anymore."

Joe was distraught. His nerves were as frayed as mine at this point. We had both been through an agonizing ordeal, watching her mind slowly go into oblivion. The outbursts and her refusal to go was the last straw for him. I knew more than anything Joe worried about my state of mind.

"No I promised her I would never put her in a home. She told me if I ever did that she would never forgive me. She told me she would never want to see me again." By now, I was out of control but the time had come to make the most difficult decision of all. I knew it, but I could not accept it. I knew Mom would never forgive me. Never.

CHAPTER 11

Joe called my brother Robert and attempted to explain what was happening. My brother owned his own business and told us that he had just moved and was right in the middle of major reorganization issues. Joe did not want to listen to him. He was so worried about my state of mind and my mother that he could not think straight. We had been keeping far too much information about Mom's illness from him. I know Robert had no idea of Joe's frame of mind, nor did Joe consider Roberts. Robert agreed to come out to Utah on the next plane. We would decide at that point what we needed to do.

Later I would come to realize we nearly put my brother out of business by forcing him to come then. We had no idea how serious things were with him. We would also find out that he and his wife had discussed having Mom stay at their place for awhile. That would have been very difficult for them with their work and family responsibilities. The problem is that we never discussed it. My brother and I never really addressed the issue of Mom's future care. Joe and I did not know about these issues until the time came to address special care for Mom. I believe we were all in denial.

Robert arrived the next day. We took Mom to day care, or I should say she insisted on going. While she was in day care, we discussed the issues and began looking around for an Alzheimer Care Facility. Few Alzheimer facilities existed In Utah at the time. They had homes for the elderly but they did not have staff trained to care for Alzheimer's patients. We did not like what we saw. They did not have areas for different levels of the disease. This was a problem because those in the final stages are just pitiful. I did not want her exposed to that, even if she did not understand more than half the time. Mom still had lucid moments when she did understand.

Both Robert and Pam were biomedical engineers. When we arrived home, Robert called his wife, as she had been looking into facilities in Wisconsin where they lived. Since they do so much geriatric testing out there, they had many facilities for the elderly, including AD-care facilities. Pam said she would continue looking and checking things out.

Pam is a very intelligent woman. Her skill in medicine, and understanding of where to go for assistance, came as a God send in this situation. She knew all the right questions to ask, and all the right people to see; she always seemed to find answers to whatever questions came up. I always admired her abilities. If it had not been for her during that time, I do not know what any of us would have done.

Later that day Pam called with information about a place that had an opening. The facility had levels of care; Mom would have her own room and could put her own things in it. She would also have her own shower and bathroom. The place was bright and cheerful with continuous activities for the patients. This is very important because AD patients need to be prompted to do things. They lose their initiative to work on their own. Group activities help keep them involved in life. The staff would also care for her health and personal care needs.

We decided to let Pam enroll her. Robert said he would just go ahead and take her back with him even though she would not go into the facility for a few weeks. Just as in the Neighborhood House, she had to complete all the paperwork and exams needed to place her properly.

When Mom arrived home, we told her she was going to stay with Robert for a while. She seemed pleased. I had already put all her paperwork and funds together for Robert. Her checkbook was a mess. I told him what had happened and just handed him a pile of papers she had in her room along with the bonds, Certificates of Deposit, checkbook and savings book. I had no idea what else he might find in them.

Robert said he would probably have to get a Power of Attorney so he could handle all of the financial issues. I told him as much as I could about her pension checks. He said Pam could take care of everything, and I agreed. She was and still is an accounting genius. I told him I would get Mom's medical and dental records sent to her new doctors as soon as possible.

Once we made the decision, Joe said he would rent a truck and move the rest of her things from Utah to Wisconsin as soon as possible. This meant she would have them when she moved into the facility. We all knew it would be better if she had her own things with her. The adjustment would be difficult enough.

Before he left, Robert took time to see Tonya's new baby. It was a sad day because Mom did not seem to recognize anyone including the baby that day. I think she was still worn out from lack of sleep during the birth.

Our home had been for sale for nearly two years but we had not had any luck selling it. We had taken it off the market right before Tonya's wedding. With all the problems with my mother we had decided to wait to put it back on the market.

As we were about to leave to take my mother and brother to the airport, an elderly couple drove into the driveway and asked if the house was still for sale. We told them it had been off the market for some time, but we might be interested in selling. The couple had advised us that they had seen our home when it was on the market and really liked it. They had just sold their home and some property and wanted to buy our house for cash right away. After explaining that we were on our way to the airport, they agreed to contact us later that day.

Joe and I could not believe our ears. We had tried to sell for over two years with few offers, now this. I did not know if we could handle another major event in our lives but the house was too much for us to maintain. It was big and had an acre of property. Now that the children were not there to help, upkeep had been very difficult.

I knew that I could not think about anything but Mom's leaving at that point. It would be for the last time. If she knew that we planned to place her in a Alzheimer's Care Facility once she arrived at Robert's home, she would never forgive me. What I was doing to her was her worst nightmare. During the fifteen years she lived with us, Mom often told me that if we ever put her in a home, she would never forgive me. She said that she would never want to see me again, and that she would no longer have a daughter. I gave her and Robert a hug and kiss good-bye. When I looked into Mom's eyes, I could tell she did not know what was about to happen to her. It nearly killed me to see that blank expression in her eyes. I felt so dishonest about not telling her everything about the trip she was making with Robert.

Joe and I watched the plane take off with our heads bowed. I cried for days afterward. I should have been relieved, but I was not. I worried about her all the time. Even when Pam called to tell us the doctor confirmed the diagnosis of Alzheimer's disease, I did not feel any less ashamed for placing her in a care facility. She was admitted into the facility in two weeks. I called often to see how things were going and could tell by my brother's voice that he was angry with me. Pam finally told me about Robert's business and how he did not know if he could save it. I knew they blamed us. I also knew that I was the most horrible person in the world or at least that is how I felt.

We should have had continual open communication with Robert throughout Mom's illness. Instead we tried to protect him against what we could see was happening to her. Joe and I knew that explaining what we were living through would be too difficult. Later I realized that Robert's family also had issues that we were unaware of. Like our mother, we all kept the bad things bottled up inside, causing many hard feelings later.

The pleasant couple did return to inspect our home once more before they made an offer. They could tell we were upset over the situation with my mother and said that they would return in a few days. They looked through the house and left. Joe and I discussed the idea of selling, and decided that a smaller place would remove a huge burden from us.

When the couple returned, we worked out a deal and signed a contract. We explained that we had to pack up Mom's things and move them to Wisconsin before we could leave the house. They were very understanding and agreed on time limits we set. So now, we had to pack Mom's stuff, pack our stuff, buy a new place, and move. When I look back on this time, I know God gave me all these things to keep me busy, and it worked. I was really busy.

I packed Mom's things. It was important to me that her surroundings be as familiar as possible for those times when she had memory flashes. I took great care in wrapping her special figurines and items precious to her. With each item, I cried a river of tears. As I packed her family pictures, memories filled my head. Sadness and tremendous guilt, overcame me.

Each time I talked to Pam, I could see that Joe and I could never have given Mom the great care that she was receiving with Robert and Pam. I knew Robert and Pam had the medical knowledge to deal with any issues that might arise. Mom would get new medications as they became available; some helped a little, some had side effects. Their knowledge of the subject far outweighed what little Joe and I knew. She was better off there, but my guilt bag continued to fill up.

Joe asked my oldest son Josh to help him drive the truck to Wisconsin. Mom's stuff nearly filled the truck. They had a terrible trip, with a bad snowstorm as they drove over the Rocky Mountains. They had hoped to drive straight through but ended up stopping for the night. The snow stopped and the roads were cleared off enough by morning for them to continue. When they arrived, Mom did not recognize Joe or Josh and was afraid of them. All they could do was unload her things and leave.

While Joe was away, I found a condominium I liked. When he returned, we went to see it together. Joe liked it as much as I did so we made an offer that the owners accepted. Since before Joe left, I had been packing and deciding what to do with years of accumulated junk. That was difficult, too. I came across more memories of the children, of my mother, of the family together. My living in an empty nest and now worrying about Mom depressed me further. On top of so many close relatives dying, my children leaving, and my mother's disease, we were now selling the house where my children grew up. These losses were tearing at the very fabric of my soul.

We finally moved into our new place. It was just the right size for the two of us, and we had extra room if the children came to visit. I should have been having fun fixing it up to suit our new lifestyle but I had this void in my heart. I had good and bad moments, but tried to keep busy and not think about Mom.

I often sent her cards with hand-painted drawings or beautiful scenes drawn on them. I knew she probably did not know from where or from whom they came, but I thought she might enjoy the pictures. She loved sweets so I sent her candy every once in awhile. Calling her was useless; she did not know who I was or what I was saying most of the time. I had to allow Robert, Pam, and their children to care for her now. It was so hard to let go, not only of my mother but of the rest of my family. Her brother and sister seemed to disagree with our putting her in a home. I knew Robert and his family were angry with us. My mother's family had always been very close despite the distance we lived from each other. Now I felt isolated. The life I once knew was gone. My aunts and uncle never actually said anything to make me believe they were angry; it was just a feeling I had that was based on my personal guilt.

So often I felt my family had disowned me. I never blamed them. I believed that I deserved it. I could not take care of Mom after all she had done for my family and me. My brother, his family and her sister and brother were in the same denial that we had been in for over a year. I felt an emptiness that would not leave for a long time.

CHAPTER 12

It was October of 1993, and I rarely heard anything about my mother since my brother moved her to Wisconsin, and I felt I did not have the right to ask. Robert and I scarcely spoke; Pam would call if there were any issues that needed to be addressed. She said that the doctors had tried different medications but did not go into what they were. She also told me that she had adjusted pretty well to her new surroundings. On special occasions they brought her to their home and sent me photographs that I treasured. I continued to send Mom cards and candy. I had no idea if she even knew what the pictures on the cards were, but I felt I had to do something to keep in touch with her. No matter what happened, my mother was always on my mind.

That month Joe received the call he had been dreading. His father had passed away. We packed and took the first plane out to Florida. His mother was so sad. It broke our hearts to see her looking so lost. They had been together for fifty-three years. Joe handled everything and took the burden off his mother and his sisters. I knew Joe was feeling much more than he let on. He, too, had learned how to keep his emotions bottled up and did it well. Salvador's death hit me hard too. He had been so good to the children and me. It felt like we were losing everyone in our families. Joe's uncle had died earlier that same year. It was not an easy time but we got through it for his mother. I returned home about a week before Joe. He stayed to help his mother complete her paperwork.

After the funeral, Joe and I returned to work, and we began to hear rumors about a major reorganization. Everyone worried about their jobs, including us. We knew something was about to happen but had no idea what. At the time, I was a Team Leader over Computer Operations. My staff was beginning to panic. For the second time in two years, the employee's jobs were in jeopardy. Unfortunately, I did not know any more than my staff did, but because I was in management, they expected me to know everything.

Then the day arrived which everyone had been dreading. Many people I had worked with for years were let go. I sat and waited for them to call my name. Every time someone was called in to the office, that person was gone. He or she would come out of the office and start packing. It was another loss in my life, one that left me feeling guilty about not losing my job. I also felt conscience-stricken about being glad that neither Joe nor I lost our jobs. None of my staff was let go and that helped, but many of my peers were gone. Even the desk next to mine was empty now.

At the time of the firings, Joe worked as a System's Security Administrator. As they called the individuals into the office, Joe had to delete their computer IDs from the systems. These were his friends and coworkers. It nearly destroyed him.

Later that day, the Vice President came around to talk to some of the remaining staff. He made the mistake of stopping at Joe's desk to ask, "So what do you think of the reorganization?" Joe proceeded to tell him in no uncertain terms. I was sure the V.P. would fire him, but Joe was a valued employee at the time and kept his job. I have to give him credit for speaking his mind. I do not think he would have said any of it if he had not been under the strain of living with an Alzheimer's patient. Joe, my rock, felt overwhelmed, too.

Joe was called on the carpet for his remarks about how he felt the company had no loyalty to those who helped build it. The V.P. put Joe in charge of Disaster Recovery as punishment for speaking his mind.

Later, we discovered that Joe loved doing Disaster Recovery. I told Joe I was proud of him sticking up for everyone. The word was out with his peers and he was the company hero. He said what everyone else wanted to say but feared the reprisal that Joe received.

To top it all off, a problem individual came to work on my shift. She had been on several other shifts and had a bad reputation. I felt that maybe I could start fresh with this person as I had had no previous contact with her. I would mentally erase the things I had heard about her and act like she was someone I met for the first time. It seemed the fair thing to do.

This strategy seemed to work for several months until changes began to take place. We went through the mass firings and the implementation of several new management dictates including a new dress code. That started the downward spiral. Sally, the company troublemaker, felt that management was being unfair. She ranted and raved and started causing problems for both her co-workers and me. Our well organized shift, that had always worked like a well-oiled machine, was breaking down.

My illness worsened. I had trouble breathing and my cough was so bad that one night I felt like I was having a stroke. At 4:00 a.m. Joe took me to the emergency room where they diagnosed me with pneumonia. That kept me out of work for almost a week, which was very unusual for me. I rarely got sick and rarely gave in to any illness or injury, but since my mother left I had become ill frequently. This time, I did not even want to get out of bed. I thought of Mom the entire time. I remembered how she would always care for me when I was little and wondered how much she hated me now. I prayed she was doing all right. I worried about my brother's business, how much he hated me. Most of all, I thought about how much I hated myself.

Even after I started feeling better physically, my mental health was terrible. I had trouble dealing with the smallest things at work. I rarely procrastinated but now, I could barely perform my daily duties. Not only did I not want to go to work, but I did not want to go home. Life, overall, became unbearable.

Several times over that year I had considered ways to kill myself. At least I once felt I was doing something good at work. My people counted on me to work with them and make the business run well. Now I did not feel that way. I submitted a request to be placed back into a technical position because I did not feel I was doing a good job as manager anymore. Now I wanted to be left alone and resented it when others dumped their problems on me. Tasks I once viewed as a challenge now overwhelmed me. My asking for a transfer should have given my management a hint that something was terribly wrong with me, but it did not.

It became my belief that no one but Joe cared and he would be so much better off without me. I wondered every day what it would be like for my family if I developed Alzheimer's disease. Discussing this problem at work was not an option. If I ever made a mistake, they might think I had Alzheimer's disease, too. I was especially paranoid after they let so many people go and Joe almost lost his job.

I worked in a fog for several months, patiently waiting to be taken out of my position and put back into a technical one. Nothing happened. During that time, I had one employee become ill and rushed to the hospital, another had an anxiety attack, and a third tried to commit suicide. The stress on the employees was beginning to show. I think my management believed I was just going through a rough time with these employees getting sick and with the known trouble maker. While those problems did not help my situation, they were not the cause. I was tired of life. Everything overwhelmed me. When I was at home, I cried all the time. At work, I barely made it through the day. I was a great actress and could put on the fake front very well. No one knew I really wanted to die.

Before everything happened to my mother, it had been a joy to have friends over. Now I dreaded anyone coming to visit. Simple tasks became more than I could handle. I felt like I could barely move sometimes. I just wanted to fall asleep and never wake up. As time went on, I became more despondent. I felt as if I was falling off a cliff and just waiting to hit bottom. Nothing was fun anymore, and I thought everyone would be better off if I were gone.

After one incident with the troublemaker at work, I came home and cried for hours. Joe asked what in the world was the matter with me lately. In a hysterical ranting, I said what had been on my mind for a long time. "I want to die. No one would miss me. My whole family hates me now. My mother would disown me for putting her in a home. Who would care?"

"What about me? I would be lost without you." He held me close as he spoke.

"You would get over it and be much better off without my constant whining, and what if I get Alzheimer's some day? Do you want to go through that again? I'm no good to anyone anymore. Besides, you can't count on me. I told Mom I would never put her in a home. Now look where she is. Did I live up to my promise?" I meant every word. That night I cried for over an hour in his arms. He knew something was very wrong. Unfortunately, Joe had no idea what it was or how to deal with it.

They had called me to Human Resources about my request. The manager asked me if this problem employee was the reason I wanted to leave. I told him that was only a small part of it. For the first time, I actually broke down while talking about it. I told the H.R. Manager that I was having difficulties at home, problems that had caused me emotional distress. I felt like a fool. Now even my eminent professional facade was going down the tubes. I wished more than ever I was dead, away from all this. This day should have been a clue to H.R. that I was in trouble emotionally. Again, nothing changed.

About a month later, an issue arose with the troublemaker. I then tried to resolve it with her and with H.R. Sally called me to her work area. A director in another department happened to be working on the color printer in our area. Sally proceeded to rant and rave, then make a comment about what a terrible team leader I was. The director just stood there in shock. The employee had totally humiliated me, but I did not want to create a scene. Finally I said, "You will have to take this up with Human Resources," and I walked away. My entire body was shaking. I tried to call someone in H.R. but had to leave a message. I hung up and practically ran to my boss's office. I knew he was out of town and I could collect myself there. I rushed past the secretary, closed the door to the office, and totally broke down. I do not remember much after that. What I do remember is almost like an out-of-body experience. I felt like that person who was always in control looking down at a whimpering childlike figure. I remember the secretary came in to check on me and found me with my head in my lap, crying like a baby. I asked her to call Joe, and she did. He had her call H.R. and the on-sight psychologist.

Once Joe came in the door from his office, he heard the H.R. representative asking me questions. My words must have been muffled because I remember I kept hearing the same questions repeated. Joe knew from past problems what had caused this dilemma. When the psychologist came in, he immediately cleared the room. He asked me a few questions that I could barely answer. I just remember bits and pieces of that conversation. I know that once we were alone, I told him I wanted to die. I asked him to leave and told him I could not take any more of this life. It took three hours but somehow he was able to get me to the point where I was calm enough to go home.

The company psychologist gave me the number where I could receive the help I needed. I knew I had some type of breakdown, and I knew I needed help. I could no longer deal with life on my own terms, and I was out of control. I agreed to go and get help.

PART III

HITTING BOTTOM

CHAPTER 13

In August of 1993, I attended my first counseling session. At this point I was in a haze. I did not know or care where I was. Not only did I not want to talk to this stranger, but I did not even want to be there at all. Joe had come with me and held my hand as we sat silently in the waiting room. A woman, close to my age, walked up and introduced herself to us. She asked to see me alone. I went in with my "be kind to strangers" attitude and we chatted for a few minutes before she gave me a questionnaire to fill out. I found it difficult answering the questions because it asked very sensitive questions about so many feelings that had been going through my head over the past year. There were questions about extreme sadness, crying all the time, and even suicide. Thinking about all these feelings put me in an even more unsettled state of mind. After I completed the form, she asked me some questions. After about the third question, I broke down and could not stop crying. She looked at me in shock and said, "You are a real pro at putting on that happy face, aren't you? You've had years of practice." I knew for the first time that someone could see through to the real me. It was disconcerting and all I could do was sob uncontrollably and feel like a fool.

She said it was obvious to her, from all my symptoms and state of mind, that I was suffering from severe depression. I had hit bottom with the breakdown that I had had at work. We discussed putting me on medication for depression. I was totally against it at first. I had taken Valium years before and suffered a blackout, so the thought of taking similar medicine scared me. She explained to me that severe depression is a chemical imbalance in the brain and that medication had changed drastically over the years. She recommended two books on the subject. I did not have the energy to argue anymore. I agreed to see my doctor and get the books and prescription. Actually I just did not care and wanted this to be over.

After the session, she wrote a note that said I needed to take an extended leave of absence from work. I also needed to have a complete physical. She wanted to see me three times a week until I started to feel results from the medication.

The first two weeks of these sessions consisted of her asking me questions about my life, I would cry uncontrollably and then she would ask more questions. I never realized all the pent-up feelings I had. It had started with my father's death, feeling guilty over not being a good enough mother, and on and on until all the guilt I felt over my mother, and finally the loss of enthusiasm for my job.

After I had been on Zoloft for four weeks, something began to happen to me. The medication seemed to bring me out the fog a little. My energy level increased. Between the medication, exercise, and change of eating habits, I started to feel human again. I knew I had a long way to go, but I could see a light at the end of the tunnel.

Joe had also been going to counseling. At first we went separately, then we went together. We gained great insight into how we interacted with each other. He especially began to see why I never shared certain aspects of my life with him. Then I began to open up to Joe. Things I had never talked about were coming out. Joe also had had a physical and been put on Zoloft. He had been coming home every night for months and falling asleep, then going up to bed and sleeping again. We did not know those were signs of depression, too.

Together we began to see each other in an entirely new way. I had to practice forgiving myself and leaving my guilt behind me. One of the best books I read during this time helped me get through this and gave me a mirror to see myself. The name of the book is I'M A DAY LATE AND A DOLLAR SHORT AND IT'S OKAY! by JoAnn Larsen. I still refer to it today.

When Joe and I began to talk about our lives and the path we were taking, he asked me what would I want to do if I could do anything. I thought for a moment and said, "I would like to take some classes and attempt a career in writing." Since I was on the medication, I had been catching up on my reading for pleasure and had begun writing poems and essays. This seemed to be a catharsis for me, but more than that, I loved doing it. I could spend hours in front of the computer and never realize that so much time had elapsed. The words seemed to flow from me like a waterfall. Joe looked me squarely in the face and asked if I were willing to take a chance. I said yes. That started what I call my rebirth. I realized how lucky I was to have a husband who, not only supported me in everything I did, but who was willing to work harder to allow me to pursue my dream.

I began to read for pleasure once again. Over the years, I had read mostly dry technical material and had been too tired to read for personal enjoyment. When I began to feel better, I think I read a hundred books. I had forgotten just how much fun it is to be in another world, a world of make-believe. I read books that I enjoyed at first, then things to help me learn the writing craft. I joined an on-line Writer's Club and took some classes.

After careful consideration, Joe and I made a major decision. I decided not to return to my job. I spoke to my boss who told me that they were going to cut another position in the Team Leader area. They had chosen one of my peers. I asked if I could leave and eliminate that postion. I told him I did not feel up to coming back, and I certainly was not ready for management responsibilities. I wrote up a request, he accepted it, and I quit my job of seventeen years.

I felt good that I had saved someone else's position at the same time. This was a major step in my life. I had been earning $45,000 a year, and now I had no income. It is funny, though, that I was not even scared. I had always said that I could contribute by working a temporary job if need be, and I did occasionally. It was fun being on the other end of things for a change. If I wanted to, I could complain about management. Still, after being in management, I could see their side of things.

I encountered another surprise. I actually enjoyed domestic life. When I worked outside the home I did not have the time or energy for domestic chores. Now I love cooking a big holiday meal for the family, and it usually turns out quite good.

For the next three years, I built a new life for myself. A few of my articles were published, and I wrote some children's books, a non-fiction novel, and two science-fiction novels. I came out of my fog and began to function. Issues remained but I had started to heal. Writing gave me a sense of self-worth that I had been lacking. It was also a great feeling to work from home. I had control over my own work environment. Many of my writings have been a release from the emotional bondage I had held myself in for many years. I realize that I could not have done it without the medication and release from work pressures, but each day I learned something new about myself.

Writing has not been an easy thing. I have had to study, read and take classes. The women in the America Online Writer's Club have inspired and supported me through every twist and turn in my new career. Every day as I sit at the computer, I wonder if anyone enjoys doing their job as much as I do. I am still a starving artist/writer, but I have made progress.

The most satisfying thing I have done recently was sending some of my poetry and essays to my eighty-three-year-old mother-in-law. She and her friends have enjoyed them so much that they recently made up a binder filled with my poems and sent them to their family members. It touched me more than anything had in a very long time. I also enjoyed writing poems for my best friend to give to her daughter at her wedding. Most recently I wrote a poem that was read at my son's wedding. I find that the pleasure of making someone feel good is better than an actual paying job. We are all so stressed these days that we need to find peace in something we do. I find it in my writing.

Joe also became a new person. He was laughing again. He no longer slept all the time when he was home, and he enjoyed his job for the first time in a long time. That V.P. who thought he was punishing Joe by changing his job did him a huge favor. It is funny how things happen; they had to replace him with two people.

For the next three years, Joe and I began to live again. After about a year, neither of us needed to continue the medication. We maintained our exercise program, ate a balanced diet, and were more relaxed.

Joe decided he needed to change jobs, too. After twenty-seven years with the same company, he resigned and instead took a similar job with a different company. Since then he continues to advance in his career and, best of all, he is content.

Recovery was a slow and sometimes difficult process. Joe and I worked together to overcome our guilt, anxiety and sadness. In my heart, I know that if I had not had the breakdown at work when I did, I would not be here today. I was on my way out of this world. It took me a long time to forgive that troubled employee who caused me to lose control. I have come to realize she saved my life. How could I feel ill will toward her?

My children were so understanding, supportive and helpful during this time. They would call or come over to spend quiet time with me whenever they could. The most wonderful thing that happened is that I enjoyed my children and granddaughter again. They were still the same wonderful family I had always had, but now I could see that. My mind had become clear again.

PART IV

CROSSING OVER

CHAPTER 14

In February of 1996, I received a call that my mother was in the hospital with a cerebral hemorrhage. I contacted my children and made flight arrangements to fly to Wisconsin. My son Matt was living in California at the time and offered to fly out with me. We were on our way in a matter of hours. I did not think about what had happened in the past, I did not think about Mom not wanting to see me. I just knew I had to be there. I knew she probably would not even know me, but none of that was important now.

Wedged between the window and a sweaty large-shouldered man in a suit, nothing seemed real anymore. Memories pounded through the fog in my head. Some brought me to a brighter time, days of taking my sons to baseball games, attending school programs, and many happy holidays. Remembering those days saddened me. I quickly turned my thoughts to the book I brought. The words on the page began to blur from the tears filling my eyes.

A woman with snow-white hair sitting in front of me began tugging at the headrest on her seat. I asked if I could help her and together we pushed the seat up so it fit behind her head comfortably. If only I could have helped my mother more. I had always been the strong one in the family. Not this time. Did I ever really admit to the illness that took over her mind and her spirit, now her body? I do not think so. If I were to admit it, I would have to accept the fact that much of her remaining time was lost to this awful disease. It took away time we could have spent together becoming closer.

I closed the book and watched the clouds rolling like a witch's brew around the plane. They reminded me of the turbulent times that Mom and I had to endure during the later phases of the disease that had stolen her from me. Then I lacked the strength to care for her. No matter how much therapy I had been through, I still felt I had turned out to be a terrible daughter. She was right. I had let her down. All those negative thoughts and guilt came rushing back to haunt me.

The man next to me finally relented and changed places with Matt. Since we had bought our tickets in such a hurry, we were not able to have our seats together. When I first sat down, I asked the man if he would consider changing places with my son, but he did not like the location of Matt's seat and refused. I did not have the energy to argue. Once Matt sat with me, I knew he would try to keep my mind off the hell we were about to encounter.

When we arrived in Chicago, we had to take a small shuttle plane to Madison. The noise in the plane made it difficult to hold a decent conversation, so my son read a magazine and dozed off and on. As I watched him sleep, I remembered the many things Mom and I had done with the boys. We had especially loved attending Josh and Matt's basketball games. We would cheer and worry about their feelings when they lost a game. I would try to keep those good times in my memory now.

Normally riding in a small plane like this would have scared me to death, but today it just did not matter. The plane finally landed. My son and I retrieved our bags and deplaned. He helped me keep my sanity that day. I had never been so grateful as when he had agreed to make the trip with me. Robert and other members of the family barely spoke to me since putting our mother in the Alzheimer's Care Facility. It would be a difficult meeting.

I dreaded seeing them, almost feared it, but I had to be there for Mom and for myself. I felt that my being there could take part of the burden off my brother and his family. It was the least I could do since I had nearly ruined his business.

I was grateful to have Matt with me. He is a charismatic, fun young man. He covered his sorrow with lighthearted conversation. I knew he had a heavy heart, too, but he did for me what I had done for my mother during my father's illness. Whenever I looked at him, I remembered those sweet words and kisses he gave Mom every night before she went to bed. Her face would light up with this small gesture. It had been the best part of her day, and it made me sad to think about it. I did not want him to hold in his feelings like I had done so often in my life.

When Matt and I arrived at the hotel, we did not even take the time to unpack but immediately took the shuttle to the hospital. As I turned the corner nearing my mother's room, I could see Robert standing near the nurse's desk. I was stunned when he hugged me. I could feel myself shaking from relief. Matt smiled, knowing what hell I had been going through about that meeting. Robert told me that our mother had had a cerebral hemorrhage. The bleeding in her brain was so extensive that they felt she would not survive very long. I could tell he was beside himself with worry. The weight of this had fallen on him and his family. Suddenly, I was glad I had come. Even if he did not know it, I could help. Although I knew my being there could not make up for all the problems I had caused, at least it would give them a chance to take time for their children and business. Knowing that Mom would not have to be left alone would surely be a relief to them, and it was wonderful seeing my sweet niece and nephew after such a long time.

A person cannot be prepared to see their mother in that condition. As we walked into her room, she looked like she was asleep. Robert told me she would not wake from the coma. I could tell he had not had any sleep for some time. I told him that we could stay in shifts so he could be with his young children and wife. He seemed relieved. Matt and I would stay until dinner and Robert and Pam would return later.

Matt and I sat next to Mom and held her hands. The nurse said they believed the patient somehow knows that there is someone there. I knew this was difficult for Matt. He was so young that he had never been around someone this ill, especially someone close to him. We talked, cried and prayed for her.

When my brother returned, we talked and tried to pretend Mom could hear everything. It was one of the strangest times of my life. Finally, I told my brother we had come there to give him a chance to do whatever he needed for his family and job. For the first time in a long time, I felt I had made the right decision in coming to be with Mom. I also asked Matt to go back to the hotel and call Joe, Tonya and Josh to let them know what was going on. He agreed and I knew he was relieved to take a break from the sadness.

Once Matt and my brother left and I was alone with Mom, the past few years of depression and guilt I had felt came to the surface. I felt like an alcoholic who just fell off the wagon. When the nurse came in to move her, she could tell, I was in terrible shape. Before we enrolled my mother in the Alzheimer's Care Facility, I had rarely been able to show my emotions in public. When the nurse left the room, I held Mom's hand and laid my head on her bedside and cried so hard my head hurt. When Robert returned, I went to the hotel for a while. I made calls to Joe and the children, had dinner with Matt, and tried to sleep but could not.

The next day a nurse, who took care of Mom in the Alzheimer's Care Facility, came to visit her. After seeing me with her, she took me to the hall away from my mother. She told me a little about how Mom had been since moving into the facility. The nurse said she was a feisty woman despite her disease. The nurse also told me not to feel guilty, and that my mother needed special care at the point when she came to the home.

She said too many daughters, sons, and other relatives cannot come to grips with putting a parent in a home. Something else she said to me hit home that day. I started to realize what we did was not all bad. The nurse told me that when family members decide to be the sole caregivers of Alzheimer's patients, they are not always aware of what they can require. The caregiver may lack the proper training to care for their parent, and later they may even come to resent or even hate, their parent.

This made sense to me. We, as children, can rarely accept what a parent says to us without taking it as their child. Many times, I felt like she hated me. I knew I should not feel that way. It was the disease talking, not my mother, but I never could really separate the two. It was years before I overcame the depression caused by caring for my mother. After talking to my mother's visitor, I sat by the bed and asked Mom to forgive me for not being strong or knowledgeable enough to take care of her. I knew what her visitor had said made sense, but my guilt would not go away.

The next few days at the hospital were horrible. Even though I knew better, every little move, reflex or blink of an eye made me wonder if she would come back. It never happened. She began to get worse. Her vital signs changed and every noise or motion seemed to bring her closer to death. She seemed to begin to struggle for breath and to swallow. The nurses had to come in often and move her around and even use a machine to suck out excess saliva since she could not swallow well. It was difficult beyond words watching her go through all this.

Matt had returned to California after three days. Joe sent me a dozen beautiful roses and a teddy bear for our anniversary. He will never know how much that meant to me. I missed Joe so very much during that time, but I was glad to be in the hotel alone. I could hug that bear and cry to my heart's content and no one would be the wiser. I still cherish that stuffed bear today. Of all the stuffed animals that my granddaughter has, she always wants to play with that bear when she visits. It is as if she knows that bear has special meaning.

The time came when the hospital said that they could not keep Mom there any longer. They were going to have to send her to a nearby nursing home. I wondered how long she could go on like this. What a strong constitution she had. Even as sick as she was, she did not want to let go.

That same day my brother's priest came in to say some prayers and give her a blessing. Mom always said she wished she had more faith because then she would not be so afraid of death. I thought about the irony of the situation. She did not want to die, and just a few years ago I longed for death.

When the day arrived for my mother to be moved to the nursing home. My sister-in-law, Pam, who had taken care of all the necessary paperwork for Mom to stay in the Alzheimer's Care Facility knew just what to do. Pam was blessed with a wonderful talent for working with the bureaucratic entanglement of medical, legal and governmental red-tape. Joe and I had had great difficulty trying to figure out Mom's government benefits, health insurance, medicare, income tax, and other intricate details we knew nothing about. We could not even imagine how to do all that Pam did for Mom.

I sat in the office with Robert, Pam, and the woman who arranged to move my mother from the hospital to the nursing home. My head was swimming. The thoughts of moving her in the condition she was in ripped at my very soul. I knew the hospital could not keep her in a room forever, but it was so hard to take.

I also knew my time and money were running out. I had been in a hotel for more than seven days and paid for my son and myself to fly to Wisconsin. I also knew when the time came that Mom did pass away, she had arrangements to be buried with my father in Arlington Cemetery in Virginia. My husband and I would fly from Utah and stay with friends there, but that was going to be very expensive, too. I hated myself for thinking of money at a time like this. How cold could I be?

By the time we finished the paperwork, Mom was in her new room at the nursing home. Next to her was a woman in her nineties. I wondered what was going through her mind as she watched my mother. I tried to talk to Mom's roommate, but she just sat there without responding. My brother and his wife stayed until they had to pick up their children at school. Their priest stopped by and asked if he could do anything. I remembered how much my mother loved the 23rd Psalm. I asked him if he could say that prayer for her, and he did. He left his Bible for me to use while I was with her. I was very grateful for his thoughtfulness.

That evening was my niece Jolynn's birthday. We took time out to have a nice dinner and cake to celebrate with her. It felt so good to be with Jolynn and Ian. It helped having the resilience of children around during such a troubling time. For that night, we all did what we knew Mom would want us to do. We celebrated Jolynn's life and time together as a family once again.

The next day it was back to reality. I sat by Mom's bed and read aloud from the priest's Bible and talked about old times. The quiet woman in the room with my mother was peeking around the curtain. My brain was on overload, my emotions right near the edge. The experience had become surreal, as if I were someone else, watching all this from above myself. I told my mother I had to leave her, that I would be flying back to Utah the next morning. It was the most difficult thing I had to do since I said goodbye to her at the airport when she was going to be put in the Alzheimer Care Facility. Deep in my heart, I knew it would be the last time I would see her alive. I cried and cried until my brother helped me walk out of the hospital. I tried to keep my emotions in check so the children did not get upset. Once back in my room, I must have cried for two hours before I finally fell asleep. I knew I was falling back into a depression but could not seem to stop it.

CHAPTER 15

The flight home was a nightmare. We had a three-hour delay due to a broken restroom. I tried to read but my mind kept returning to my mother, in her room waiting to die. The thoughts tortured me all the way home. When I deplaned, I fell into Joe's waiting arms and sobbed again.

Each morning and afternoon, I called the nursing home to see if Mom's condition had changed. I guess I hoped for a miracle but knew there would be none. I just had to feel close to her in some way. The nurses were all sweet and patient. They must have had a thousand phone calls from relatives wishing they could be there but for some reason could not.

I received the call two days after returning home. I had just finished my laundry when the phone rang. Robert said that Mom had died. I knew it was coming, but it was still a shock when it actually happened. I seemed to think she would always be there. Then suddenly she was not. I felt as if a part of me had been severed.

Joe arranged for our trip to Washington, D.C. When I called my friend, she said the room was always ready for us and told me how sorry she was about my mother.

Again, the long flight was a blur. I do not even remember it to this day. I do remember thinking about facing all those relatives who had resented me for putting her in the home. I dreaded having to talk to them or see them.

I enjoyed seeing my friend Joann after so many years. It seemed like we had just been together even though many years had gone by. I felt better for a short time; Joann always had that effect on me. We had done crazy things in our younger days. We looked at pictures and reminisced about them, then talked about our children who had since grown. After twenty years, we even had grandchildren to talk about.

Then my cousin Fran called. She tried to tell me not to feel guilty about anything, but that just made me feel even worse. I knew she was trying to help, and I was grateful when she offered to hold a buffet at her home after the funeral. I had been trying to decide what to do but wanted to wait until Robert arrived. Fran told me all my aunts and uncles knew I had had no choice. Of course I knew how they felt, no matter what she said. They would try to be forgiving, but I knew they did not agree with my decision to put her in the Alzheimer's Care Facility. At that time I tried to ignore what my relatives thought and concentrate on the funeral and saying goodbye to my mother.

It was a traditional military funeral. The soldiers carried her casket to the grave site and the priest said prayers. Here we were, some twenty years after my father's death, back at Arlington Cemetery. Mom would be placed in the same grave as my father which is what they both wanted. I hoped and prayed they were now together, watching out for each other. More than anything, I was glad that my mother no longer had to bear this terrible disease.

Joann and her husband had come to the funeral. I felt that neither of them would fully understand why I could not control my emotions. Only Joe and I knew about the horror of the past years we had spent together watching a vibrant, intelligent, woman, mother, and grand-mother lose all she had held so dear. In the back of my mind, I always tried to believe when people have Alzheimer's disease, their minds go to another dimension. It helped me to believe that in this place they feel no pain and see only angels. I guess we all do what we must to survive this terrible thing.

When I returned home, I began to feel as though I were losing my eyesight. Things were very blurry all the time. I was also thirsty all the time and urinated frequently. I finally got scared enough about my eyesight that I went to the doctor. He told me that I had developed diabetes, and that it was stress induced because of my mother's death. My father had been a diabetic. For some strange reason I felt that having diabetes was a sign that I may take after my father instead of my mother where my health was concerned, and that gave me comfort. I would die of a diabetic related problem instead of developing Alzheimer's disease like my mother. Strange how things like that go through our minds. I knew then that I did not want to die. I have far to much to live for.

EPILOGUE

I still pray a cure for Alzheimer's disease will be found soon. Four million Americans have Alzheimer's disease and nineteen million Americans say they have a family member with Alzheimer's. These statistics are staggering, and with the baby-boomers all turning fifty, it will only get worse. The burden to families, to the economy, and to the care facilities and the housing of these patients will be over-whelming.

Today, I sit at this computer and am able only to write for one half-hour at a time before my emotions take over. Every time I forget a word or blank out, I think about my mother and worry that I will be the next to develop this disease, but I do not dwell on that anymore.

Every day I thank my husband and children, who were always patient, kind and understanding during this terrible time in our lives. Without them, I do not think I would have survived.

I know how lucky I am, and I hope writing this will help others going through similar tragedies in their lives. I do not have any real words of wisdom, mostly because I do not feel I was very wise during all this. Looking back, I could have handled things better, done things different-ly, and perhaps been able to help my mother more than I did. I am not sure it would have changed anything but at least we would not have gone through this alone. Although we all have to do the best we can at the time, we have to learn to live with the consequences of our actions.

There comes a time, though, when we need to forgive ourselves in order to continue to survive this life. I think I am finally doing that by writing this book.

There are many new treatments but still no cure for Alzheimer's disease. The future looks promising. With new research in the study of DNA, I pray that a cure will be found soon.

On May 2, 1999, an article called "Scientists Seeking to Grow New Parts to Fix Disabled Brains" in **The Salt Lake Tribune** discussed cell therapy. The last paragraph said, "These scientist envision a day when repairing a broken brain will involve no transplants, no operation. Instead, it will mean triggering the brain to awaken its supply of stem cells, to grow its own spare parts, to literally fix itself." This sounds like science fiction to me but stranger things have happened. I need to hold out hope for myself and other family members who may carry this gene.

In the December 1999 **Prevention Magazine,** in the section called, *On the Horizon,* they write about a Vaccine for Alzheimer's being possible in the future. It says. "Researchers could begin human testing on a promising Alzheimer's vaccine late this year or early next year.

The vaccine prompts the immune system to destroy protein that forms destructive plaque formation in young mice and reversed plaque buildup in older mice (Nature, July 7, 1999).

If the vaccine performs well in the upcoming small-scale safety trail, it could be tested on a larger scale later, says lead researcher Dale Schenk, PhD, of the Elan Corporation, the vaccine's developer."

If individuals like Burgess Meredith, Rita Hayworth, Sugar Ray Robinson and Ronald Reagan are susceptible to this disease, we all need to be aware and educated on the subject. We need to understand the symptoms and warning signs, but more important, we need not to assume it is Alzheimer's. There are many other illnesses that can mimic Alzheimer's. Only a doctor can help lead you to the correct diagnosis. Usually a psychiatrist performs tests that tell what portions of the brain are working in a certain way. This gives them clues as to the actual problem.

I have asked my doctor to put me back on Estrogen, I take vitamin E, exercise and eat more healthy than ever before. I want to be around and know my grandchildren and perhaps even great-grandchildren. I remain hopeful that a cure seems closer than ever. Each day they are finding out new things about the Alzheimer's gene. It is projected that if the disease continues as is, by the middle of the 21st century, fourteen million will be affected.

Recently I was watching a talk show on television where they discussed how family members that care for their parents are practicing good *family values*, I feel that guilt well up inside me again. We each do what we can. Maybe it is not what society wants, or is not, *good family values*, but we each do our best. That of course is different for each situation and for each family. Every day I attempt to go on with my life. It is not always easy because I know how many others are going through the same thing I did. That is why I thought it was so important to write this book. In the beginning of this disease, I was uneducated. If this book can help one person say, "This story helped me care for my mother or father," I feel I've done something worthwhile.

To all of you, especially those not so perfect caregivers, my prayers and sympathy are with you and your families.

The End.

REFERENCES

Alzheimer's Association Web Page,
Salt Lake Tribune, Prevention Magazine

DESCRIPTION

STOLEN MEMORIES deals with the impact of being a caregiver for a parent and how it not only affects one's job and family, but also one's mental and physical health. This story deals with the guilt that caregivers often carry as the gradually have to invade their parent's privacy in order to keep them safe—everything from having to take a driver's license away, to having to put a parent into an Alzheimer's care facility. Marie encounters feelings of helplessness as she has to go against her mother's wishes in order to care for her. Later her struggles through her own dark depression as the hopeless prognosis of Alzheimer's disease takes its toll on her entire family, understands her agonizing sense that no matter what she did, it wasn't enough.

STOLEN MEMORIES deals with real issues that confront many of us. It is important that those who have been through caring for a parent with Alzheimer's disease share their stories, as these experiences may help someone recognize and deal with this disease in its early stages.

ABOUT THE AUTHOR

I wrote STOLEN MEMORIES—ONE FAMILY'S EXPERIENCE WITH ALZHEIMER'S DISEASE after my mother died from complications from Alzheimer's disease in 1996.

Although I was fortunate to have the wholehearted support of my husband, our busy life, our growing children, and the deteriorating condition of my mother (who lived with us) was overwhelming at times. I wrote STOLEN MEMORIES to give support, comfort, and hard-earned knowledge to other imperfect people who find themselves in the position of caregiver.

Changing roles with a parent can be difficult, confusing and devastating. They often overlook caregivers, but the impact upon them is greater than most realize. The guilt I felt after placing my mother into a nursing home, caused me to suffer a nervous breakdown.

I want my experiences to be a warning to others. Much of what I went through could have been avoided, if I had known the symptoms of Alzheimer's disease, if I had not tried to be Superwoman, and if I had been aware of how our childhood affect us when we become adults in crisis.

I am opening up my life, however painfully, in hopes that my experiences will avert a similar disaster in the lives of others dealing with Alzheimer's disease.

Visit the Alzheimer's Disease Caregivers Community for additional information at:

http://communities.iuniverse.com/bin/circle.asp?circleid=1506

Contact the Author

Marie Cloud
P.O. Box 18488
Kearns, Utah 84118
E-mail   mcloud@addall.com

www.ingramcontent.com/pod-product-compliance
Lightning Source LLC
Chambersburg PA
CBHW020246290526
45784CB00003B/1113